OLD RED

Pioneering Medical Education in Texas

By Heather Green Wooten

Texas State Historical Association
Denton

Number twenty-two in the Fred Rider Cotten Popular History Series

Library of Congress Cataloging-in-Publication Data
Wooten, Heather Green, 1958–
Old Red : pioneering medical education / by Heather Green Wooten.
    p. cm. — (Fred Rider Cotten popular history series ; no. 22)
Includes bibliographical references.
ISBN 978-0-87611-254-0
1. Ashbel Smith Building (Galveston, Tex.) 2. University of Texas. Medical Branch—Buildings—History. 3. University of Texas Medical Branch at Galveston—Buildings—History. 4. College buildings—Texas—Galveston—History. 5. Galveston (Tex.)—Buildings, structures, etc.—History. 6. Clayton, Nicholas Joseph, 1839–1916. 7. Medical education—Texas—History. I. Title. II. Series: Fred Rider Cotten popular history series; no. 22.
  F394.G2W66 2012
  976.4'139—dc23

                                                    2012038546

CONTENTS

ACKNOWLEDGEMENTS

THE ORIGINAL INSPIRATION FOR THIS BOOK occurred over a decade ago when, as a graduate student at the Institute for the Medical Humanities at the University of Texas Medical Branch (UTMB) in Galveston, I had the pleasure of attending classes inside the Ashbel Smith Building, fondly nicknamed "Old Red." Throughout my studies there, I felt part of a great tradition and hoped to have an opportunity to convey that spirit in some way. This book, at least in part, addresses that goal.

One of the delights of writing this book was the immense support I received from professional colleagues and friends. First of all, I am deeply grateful to Ryan Schumacher, associate editor for the Texas State Historical Association (TSHA) Press and Randolph B. "Mike" Campbell, chief historian of the TSHA for their everlasting support and confidence in my work. I also want to thank the anonymous reviewer for a critique that served to vastly enrich this narrative. I extend special gratitude to UTMB program director of Facilities Operation and Management, Robert "Bob" Brown, for taking the time to supply the latest updates on the structural status of Old Red. Other enthusiastic champions of this project include Howard Brody, director of the Institute for the Medical Humanities at UTMB; Brett Kirkpatrick, director of the Moody Medical Library; and Eddie Weller, my department chair and mentor at San Jacinto College South.

Several skilled archivists and librarians deserve special praise for their assistance on this project. The Truman G. Blocker Jr. History of Medicine Collections at the Moody Medical Library contains a wealth of information on Old Red, architect Nicholas J. Clayton, and the history of UTMB. I am especially indebted to Blocker Collections archivists Robert "Bobby" Marlin and Sarita Oertling, who put their treasure trove at my disposal. Particular gratitude is extended to Sarita for her exceptional help in sourcing many of the illustrations for this book. The Galveston and Texas History Center (GTHC) at the Rosenberg Library was another wonderful resource. My heartfelt appreciation goes to GTHC director

Casey Greene, Carol Wood, and members of the staff, who were most helpful is retrieving files and photographs for my use. I would like to extend additional thanks to the Galveston County Historical Commission for their assistance and support of this effort.

Finally, the book profited immensely from the labor and talents of key individuals. I am deeply grateful to Clare Cozad for her patient and thorough reading of multiple versions of this manuscript and her helpful critique of each. Special acknowledgement goes to Dina Boomer, whose skills in manuscript preparation, graphic design, and document formatting were essential to the completion of this book.

In addition, a special acknowledgement is extended to my grand-dog, Manny Campbell, whose canine guidance and insistence upon play and affection extended this project for months on end.

INTRODUCTION

TUCKED AWAY IN A CORNER OF THE CAMPUS of the University of Texas Medical Branch (UTMB) stands a majestic relic of an era long past. Designed by renowned Texas architect Nicholas J. Clayton and completed in 1890, the beautifully ornate, red brick Ashbel Smith Building, fondly nicknamed "Old Red," represents a remarkable page in Galveston and Texas history. Within this extraordinary building in early October 1891, a small group of visionary physicians launched the University of Texas medical program. It marked the culmination of years of effort by numerous individuals, including those of pioneer physician-educator Ashbel Smith, whose lifelong dream entailed the establishment of a university-based medical school. Today, Old Red, the premier symbol of medical education in Texas, ranks among the state's landmarks in a class alongside the Texas Capitol, the Governor's Mansion, and the Alamo.

This book will examine the life and legacy of the Ashbel Smith Building from its beginnings through the contemporary efforts to preserve it. Chapters explore the nascence of medical education in Texas; the supreme talent and genius of Old Red architect Nicholas J. Clayton; and the lives of faculty and students as they labored and learned in the midst of budget crises, classroom and fraternity antics, death-rendering storms, and threats of closure. The education of the state's first professional female and minority physicians and the nationally acclaimed work of physician-scientists and researchers are also highlighted. The spirited campaign by UTMB officials, alumni, and friends to save and restore Old Red rounds out the narrative.

Best of all, I invite the reader to step inside Old Red and mingle with ghosts of the past: to ascend the magnificent cedar staircase, wander the long, paneled hallways, take a seat for a lecture in the tiered amphitheater, or enjoy the macabre spectacle found in the old anatomy lab, where cadavers are laid out in rows and jars of pathology specimens twinkle in the sunlit space.

Chapter 1

IN SEARCH OF A
MEDICAL SCHOOL

IT WAS THE MOMENT the aged physician had long awaited. On March 30, 1881, the Texas Legislature voted to establish the University of Texas and a medical department to go with it. Almost a half century had passed since Ashbel Smith left a successful medical practice in North Carolina to pursue life in Texas. In 1837, with a medical doctorate from Yale and a year of medical study in Paris under his belt, Smith arrived at the invitation of soldier and statesman James Pinckney Henderson, befriended General Sam Houston, and was quickly appointed surgeon general of the army of the Republic of Texas. For the next fifty years, Smith followed his quest to establish educational and medical excellence in his adopted state. After decades of effort, Smith's dream of a first-class medical school in Texas had become a reality. "The Medical Department, when properly organized," the seventy-four-year-old Smith enthusiastically proclaimed, "will . . . be the leading, paramount school of Medical Instruction of the great Southwestern region of the American Union."[1] The future of the proposed medical school looked bright indeed, but many challenges still lay ahead before it would be established.

Medicine was an archaic enterprise throughout most of the nineteenth century. Traditionally taught as an art rather than as a science, medical expertise was most often acquired through trial and error on patients rather than in the medical laboratory. A physician's résumé consisted primarily of delivering babies, setting broken bones, prescribing drugs, and comforting the dying. Common plagues such as typhoid, pneumonia, tuberculosis or "consumption," and "the itch" were confronted with age-old medical "remedies" that included bloodletting, blistering, and a variety of potentially toxic potions. Patients who survived the sickbed often did so only because of a strong physical predisposition or luck rather than the doctor's care.

Insufficient medical training was part of the problem. In the mid-nineteenth century, almost anyone who aspired to study medicine could do so. School choice consisted of two categories: university or proprietary (privately owned). Both were seriously understaffed and offered a very basic curriculum, which was frequently taught by harried faculty who were poorly paid. Proprietary schools were commonly considered no more than "diploma mills." With enrollment fees often the sole resource for funding, these institutions welcomed almost any applicant who demonstrated the ability to pay the tuition and read and write. The least qualified of this lot were offered a medical degree by mail.[2]

Many aspiring practitioners sidestepped the medical school route altogether. The apprenticeship system, prevalent for centuries, enabled young men to study the art of healing for a "winter or two" under the guidance of an established practitioner. While competent practitioners emerged from this shaky system, it primarily produced masses of unqualified physicians, quacks, and pretenders. By 1850 the respect of the medical degree had so declined that some medical leaders wished to do away with it completely. In the absence—or avoidance—of medical expertise, Americans in search of medical care explored other options. Many embraced the teachings of native sects or joined health cults such as those espoused by Sylvester Graham and Bronson Alcott that created a secular religion out of trends in hygiene, diet, and bodily discipline. Others consumed patent medicines by the gallon. Daly's Aromatic Valley Whiskey for Medicinal Purposes was a favorite, as was Old Sachem Bitters and Wigwam Tonic.[3]

The best hope of young Americans for obtaining a respectable medical degree involved study abroad. Nineteenth-century European medical schools, especially those in France and Germany, strongly advocated progressive ideas and practices that left a profound influence upon their American pupils. At a celebrated Paris medical school, the École de Médicine, French physicians of international renown lectured and allowed students to accompany them on their hospital rounds. In addition to providing clinical commentary, these physician-teachers gave lectures on twenty-six medical topics, including anatomy, surgical pathology, therapeutics, diseases of women and children, and legal medicine. For American students like Ashbel Smith, the greatest contribution to come out of the Paris school was the concept that factual evidence was essential to accurate diagnosis. When a violent outbreak of cholera swept through Paris in 1832, Smith treated the sick, and in off-duty hours he performed autopsies to learn the nature of the disease. After the epidemic passed, Smith published a pamphlet that described in detail the symptoms, pathology, and treatment of the disease—all acquired through extensive study.[4]

The Germans also made great strides in medicine. Research conducted in German medical laboratories proclaimed the dawn of modern-day bacteriology and its wholesale significance to antiseptic surgery and public health. Americans studying abroad embraced the innovative skills and philosophies espoused by European physicians and eagerly applied them in their own practices upon their return to the United States. German influence upon American medicine extended beyond theory and practice. German physicians in particular received their training within the university system. Here, education and scientific advances went hand-in-hand. Physicians interested in full-time teaching and research earned the respected identity of professors. While enlightened American medical educators began to adopt German principles as early as the 1850s, the Civil War postponed genuine progress until the 1870s.[5]

Medical practice in America during the Civil War period was a profound mixture of good and bad. The first year of the war in particular highlighted the inherent disorganization and ineptitude of both Union and Confederate army medical departments. Ignorance regarding the spread of germs and bacteria caused infectious diseases to rage within the camps. Calomel, a cathartic, and tartar emetic were implemented wholesale. Regimental physicians refused to care for patients other than their own. Medical records were lost. Hospitals buckled under sudden onslaughts of the sick and wounded. The Confederate medical situation remained desperate throughout the war as the army struggled with an ever-dwindling supply of food, drugs, blankets, and other necessities.

The war also hastened medical advances. At the height of the conflict, the Union army contained approximately 11,000 physicians, while the Confederates boasted almost 6,000 medical enlistees. The best-qualified practitioners took examinations to become regimental surgeons. Many received their commissions from state governors. Experience on the battlefield in handling the knife, the saw, and the use of anesthesia (ether and chloroform) gave these physicians invaluable experience and proficiency regarding surgical care. Many began to appreciate the connection between microbes and disease. For instance, United States Surgeon General William Hammond introduced a sound system for classifying diseases, encouraged procedures to ensure better hygiene and sanitation, and demanded better record-keeping procedures as a means of improving performance. The Confederate medical situation also improved through the able leadership of Surgeon General Samuel Preston Moore, who made the best of debilitating shortages. Both armies benefited from the world's first ambulance corps.[6]

The nursing profession also received a boost. Previously, few women of means and certainly no "lady" entered the profession. Hospital nurses came from the dregs of society, most of whom, according to nursing reformer Florence Nightingale, "were too old, too weak, too drunken, too dirty, too stolid, or too bad to do anything else."[7] Nightingale's courageous and untiring efforts to alleviate suffering among the British wounded during the Crimean War (1854–56) laid the foundation of professional nursing. Upon her return to England, Nightingale established in 1860 the first secular nursing school in the world at St. Thomas' Hospital in London. These actions had a profound influence upon American women, both North and South. As the incredible carnage of the battlefield assailed their communities, women labored to alleviate the suffering around them. Union nurses Clara Barton and Mary Ann Bickerdyke as well as the Confederate Sally Louise Tompkins organized successful war hospitals in their respective regions. Programs that would teach viable nursing skills were at a premium. Many of the well-educated and administratively efficient members of the U.S. Sanitary Commission became the primary motivators behind the creation of postwar nursing schools. Invalid corps in both the North and South effectively utilized the restless energy of disabled soldiers for guard duty, nursing, and other tasks. Each of these wartime initiatives gave birth to progressive medical theories and practices.[8]

The Civil War arrived before the German medical education principles of the 1850s firmly took hold in America. Not until after the Confederate surrender at Appomattox did many American universities begin incorporating the independent medical school into their systems. Once they did, the quality of American medical instruction improved dramatically. University regents raised admission standards, expanded curriculum, and lengthened academic terms. Newly constructed facilities featured fully equipped laboratories, libraries, and other tools for scientific teaching and research. Each of these academic innovations benefited the American medical profession.

Progressive-minded Texans soon took notice. Many aspiring physicians in Texas traveled east of the Mississippi to attend one of the university medical schools. Galveston newspapers in particular featured advertisements from the University of Louisville School of Medicine, the Medical Department of the University of Nashville, and New York Medical College.[9] The academic successes of these schools captured the imagination of crusaders in the West. Before long, Texas reformers began agitating for a university medical school of their own.

This idea was not entirely new. During the days of the Texas Republic, President Mirabeau B. Lamar, a fierce advocate for public education, championed the insertion of a provision into the original state constitution of 1845 to establish a state university and medical department. Lamar's campaign quickly stalled and unfortunately remained on the legislative shelf for the next twenty years. However, a few minor attempts at medical education were made during the interim. One of particular note occurred in 1855 when Galveston physician Thomas Stanwood endeavored to make the most of the hanging of convicted murderer John Schultz. The *Galveston News* reported that, promptly after the criminal's execution, "the body was then immediately delivered into the hands of Dr. Stanwood who removed it to a convenient place for a hasty dissection" and anatomy demonstration for persons in attendance. The body, sans "cranium," was buried at the conclusion of Stanwood's lecture.[10]

It was no accident that Stanwood chose Galveston for his efforts toward medical enlightenment. From its founding, Galveston occupied a central place in conversations pertaining to medicine and health in Texas. Pioneer physicians in the early decades of the nineteenth century praised the healthiness of the island city. According to Ashbel Smith, the invigorating island sea breezes combined with warm Gulf water for bathing made Galveston the ultimate health resort. "If you have any invalids," wrote Smith to a friend in 1839, "send them among us. An abundance of seafood—an atmosphere unrivalled for balminess and salubrity—and novelty of scenes and the excitement of a virgin country are at the command of the dyspeptic. For rheumatics and consumptives the climate is particularly genial."[11] Smith's sentiments were echoed by a British diplomat on a visit to "the Island" (the shortened term for Galveston Island often used by locals and visitors) in 1841: "[P]estential [*sic*] diseases . . . so common in the West Indies, [are] here unknown . . . in a word the mildness and salubrity of the climate of this region has no equal in America."[12]

Not everyone viewed Galveston through such a wholesome lens. Stephen F. Austin noted the coastal areas of Texas appeared far less healthy than those further inland.[13] An 1837 visitor to the Island concurred, "the lower country, from the Trinity to the Colorado, is as sickly as the most unhealthful portions of Louisiana . . . The country becomes healthier at any point as you recede from [the] gulf."[14] By the 1840s, many individuals began to view Galveston not as a hub of health but a city teeming with pestilence. Swarms of mosquitoes plagued residents making it impossible to sleep without protective netting. Poor sanitation reigned and deadly diseases extracted heavy tolls, especially of children, each year. Citizens lived in fear of typhoid, smallpox, dengue fever—and the most dreaded of all—yellow fever. Prior to 1860, seven epidemics of "yellow jack" or "vomit noir" claimed over 2,300 lives. During the late summer of 1853, the disease caused an average of fourteen deaths per day. The most virulent epidemic gripped the Island in 1867, when over 1,150 succumbed out of the approximately 16,000 residents. Each repeated visit of "yellow jack" increased Galveston's reputation as a "sickly city."[15]

Galveston physicians and caregivers confronted the epidemics with a limited therapeutic arsenal. As a rule, antebellum physicians followed a medical belief system based upon maintaining a bodily equilibrium. If illness or disease upset that delicate balance, attempts were made to restore it by means of "heroic" medical procedures. Copious bleeding followed by purging highlighted the list of therapies. In cases of yellow fever, physicians advocated the lancet, mustard baths, and purgatives as necessary tools in treating the disease. While disagreements arose concerning the proper dosage, Galveston practitioners adhered to the standard procedures.[16]

Yellow fever outbreaks in Galveston fostered significant medical breakthroughs, however. During a severe yellow fever epidemic in 1839, Ashbel Smith utilized the long hours treating yellow fever patients to unravel mysteries surrounding the disease. No one knew the source of yellow fever or how it was transmitted. Many physicians believed the disease was contagious, spread directly or indirectly between individuals. Others maintained an attack of yellow fever resulted from "local" conditions such as climate, poor sanitation, and airborne effluvia. Smith supported the latter theory. He maintained meticulous medical case records and, to ultimately prove his point, operated on the bodies of nine yellow fever victims. In his report, *Account of Yellow Fever in Galveston in 1839*, the first medical narrative printed and published in Texas, Smith revealed a courageously intimate—and squirm-inducing—methodology. To prove yellow fever was not contagious, Smith freely handled diseased organs, liberally immersed his hands in black vomit and other bodily fluids, closely viewed and smelled them—even "*repeatedly tasted* the black vomit, when fresh ejected from the stomachs of the living."[17] In each instance, the doctor's health remained unscathed.

To keep the disease away from Galveston, Smith recommended the city remove filth from the streets and fill in disease-producing marshlands around the Island. Many citizens embraced Smith's theories. As the 1839 epidemic waned, patient Lucy P. Shaw proudly noted: "We are fortunate in having an excellent physician, Doctor Smith . . . I am perfectly well now and all our family are well, although we have had so many deaths in our house and the yellow fever has taken away a great many on the Island . . . Dr. Smith is perfectly well and has never had any symptoms of the disease, and if it was contagious I think he would . . . There are ten resident physicians on the Island . . . but we think we have found the best."[18] Other citizens remained skeptical that yellow fever could be controlled so easily. Until the identification of the yellow fever virus and the mosquito as the transmission source in 1902, frightened Galveston residents continued to support strict quarantine and sanitation procedures as the primary means of protection from the disease. Nevertheless, Smith's work in Galveston set a precedent for future research by medical pioneers in the realm of medicine and public health.[19]

The ongoing threat of disease in Galveston also spurred the establish-

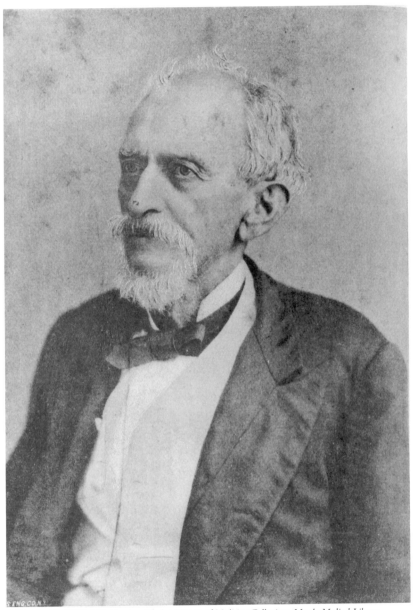

Ashbel Smith (1805–86). *Courtesy Blocker History of Medicine Collections, Moody Medical Library.*

ment of hospitals and good nursing care. No health care institutions existed on the Island before 1838. The situation changed with the onslaught of yellow fever epidemics. Many victims of yellow fever and other diseases were European immigrants newly arrived to the port city en route west. The surging caseload of indigent sick compelled Galveston officials to establish a hospital to care for them. The first hospital on the Island, the Galveston City Hospital, was a primitive affair. Located on the bay shore of the Island, approximately a mile and a half from the city, the hospital was little more than a wooden hovel. Charles Hooten, a visitor to Galveston in 1841, offered this picture: "[The hospital] stood alone in the desert dead, silent, and seemingly aloof from all living and active Christian sympathy."[20] The illustration that accompanied Hooten's stark description of the hospital featured a small, wood-frame structure set among marshes and sand dunes on the bay side of the Island. In 1845 a larger and more accessible charity hospital was constructed on Ninth and Strand Streets. Three stories tall and capable of accommodating nearly one hundred patients, the new facility was a significant improvement over its predecessor.[21]

More than twenty years after the opening of the new city hospital, a Catholic nursing order, the Sisters of Charity of the Incarnate Word, spearheaded their own charity institution. Armed with the purpose of saving bodies as well as souls, the Sisters of Charity became the most active order of Catholic nuns in pioneer medical service in Texas. Arriving from France in April 1867, the sisters, led by Bishop Claude M. Dubuis, staffed a thirty-bed facility that became the first Catholic hospital in Texas. It was fortuitous timing. In July, a raging yellow fever epidemic swept the Island filling the wards of both the Charity and Galveston City hospitals to overflowing. For five months, the sisters worked tirelessly at the bedsides of the stricken. The nurses overcame many challenges involving patients, including communication and culture shock. The French nuns labored to master, as one noted, "a fair—if not elegant—speaking knowledge" of English from their patients.[22]

In an era when most sick people received medical treatment at home, some patients balked at the ministrations of the nuns attired in strange dress and who upheld a passion for cleanliness. By the epidemic's departure in November, the sisters had closed the eyes of many victims, including one of their own: the young superior, Sister Blandine Mathelin. After a brief closure, the hospital reopened as St. Mary's Infirmary in 1869. The enterprise grew. Additional sisters arrived from France to aid in the effort. Within a few short years, the Sisters of Charity acquired an orphanage and had replaced the infirmary's frame building with two three-story, beautifully ornate brick structures (completed in 1875 and 1879, respectively) that supplied ample ward space and facilities for nursing care.[23] Through enterprise and effort, the Galveston medical community succeeded in providing care for all who needed it.

Along with a burgeoning hospital system came the first attempt to launch a medical school in Galveston. In 1855 the Methodist Episcopal Church South established a university named in honor of Bishop Joshua Soule at Chappell Hill, Texas. After the university governing board obtained a charter from the Texas Legislature, it created chairs for law, medicine, and biblical science. Sensing an opportunity, Dr. G. W. Neely proposed the creation of an affiliated medical school in Galveston. The suggestion had merit. Not only would a medical school be a prestigious plum for the Island, but as a southern institution, it could provide the experience necessary to treat diseases distinctive to the region, including dengue and yellow fever. A group of enthusiastic Gulf Coast physicians formed a committee to pursue the matter. In addition to Neely, the committee members included Ashbel Smith, William R. Smith, and Thomas J. Heard of Galveston; Professor Stone and Dr. McFarland of New Orleans; and William H. Gantt of Washington County, Texas.[24]

While hopes ran high among the committee, timing was not in their favor. Just as the project gained momentum, Texas joined fellow southern states in the secessionist cause as civil war divided the nation. Galveston felt the effects almost immediately. By July of 1861, Federal naval forces had successfully encircled the port and began to squeeze the city. Local businesses collapsed. Federal troops infiltrated the financially strapped Island. Many physicians, including members of the planning committee, were called to the battlefield. Those left behind lacked the time, resources, or energy needed to pursue the establishment of a medical school. The dream would have to wait.

Everything changed with the Confederate surrender in April 1865. Within months, the Island entered an era of sweeping prosperity. Christened the "Queen City of the Gulf," Galveston became the largest and wealthiest city in the state. Postwar Galveston embodied a mixture of the old and the new as classic southern charm blended with vigorous enterprise and capitalism. A restless, energetic migrant population poured in and out of Galveston as the Island port became the gateway to the Southwest. Half of the cotton grown in Texas was exported through the Island port while the profits funded magnificent mansions, financed insurance companies, and opened banks. A fresh, aggressive social elite sprang up in the place of the old planter class ruined by the war. Millionaires with the names of Moody, Kempner, and Sealy dominated the Island with fortunes gleaned from banking and mercantilism. On the northern end of Galveston, the Strand business district—the "Wall Street of the Southwest"—became the state's crown jewel of economic, social, and cultural activity. The Grand Opera House, built in 1894, hosted famous opera ensembles, ballet performances, and the best theatrical productions in the state. Galveston in the decades following the war also claimed many firsts for Texas. The city boasted the first national bank, the first chamber of commerce, and the first public library. It was also the home of the first electric light system, the first telephone, and the first baseball game played in the state.[25]

Physicians flocked to Galveston lured by the prospects of cash and prestige. Many hoped to profit from services rendered to the well-to-do and the rest of the twenty-thousand-plus population. Others came to attend the many indigent patients at the Galveston City and St. Mary's hospitals. These institutions, combined with an abundance of resident physicians, offered a unique, specialized environment found nowhere else in the state. According to the Galveston City Directory, over fifty physicians practiced on the Island during the Reconstruction years.[26] Establishing a medical school was just as important to post-Civil War Galveston physicians as providing medical care. With their support, the Soule University medical department, formally designated the Galveston Medical College, opened its doors in November 1865. Local medical doctors supplemented their incomes by serving on the faculty. They included Nathaniel N. Allen, Professor of Surgery; Jesse Boring, Professor of Obstetrics and Diseases of Women and Children; William H. Gantt, Professor of Physiology and Pathological Anatomy; David P. Smythe, Professor of Chemistry; Charles W. Trueheart, Demonstrator of Anatomy; John L. Watkins, Professor of Medical Theory and Practice; and John H. Webb, Professor of Materia Medica and Therapeutics. Through a series of classroom lectures and demonstrations, this body of "professors" sought to instill higher standards of medical professionalism. In order to graduate, students were required to maintain excellent attendance, demonstrate proficiency in all coursework, and regularly attend patients. A sound moral character and satisfactory technical skills topped off the list of conditions.[27]

Although dedicated instructors and students were paramount to the success of Galveston Medical College, the power behind the endeavor was Dr. Greensville Dowell, the medical college dean and professor of surgery. A graduate of Jefferson Medical College in Philadelphia, Dowell first arrived in Galveston as a Confederate Army surgeon. Even besieged in wartime, the coastal city exhibited a dynamism that Dowell could not resist. Rather than return east at the end of the war, Dowell remained in Galveston, opened a practice, and launched a mission to set the Galveston medical community apart from others in the Southwest. His track record was impressive. Within a few short years, he helped found the Galveston Medical Society, the first medical society in Texas; wrote extensively;

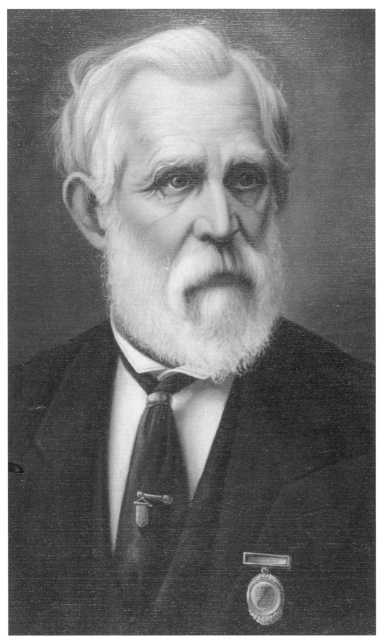

Greensville Dowell (1822–88). The first dean and driving spirit of the Galveston Medical College and Hospital, Dowell was devoted to creating higher standards of medical professionalism in Texas. *Courtesy Blocker History of Medicine Collections, Moody Medical Library.*

and published the *Galveston Medical Journal*, the first medical periodical in the state. A leading authority on yellow fever, Dowell often traveled to epidemic-stricken cities to aid in the treatment of victims. His widely read work *Yellow Fever and Malarial Diseases* (1876) includes an account of his own experiences as well as reports written by other Texas physicians.[28] Local and state recognition of Dowell's many professional contributions aided the promotion of Galveston Medical College.

Still, a variety of issues plagued the school from the start. One problem involved location. Members of the local business community balked at the college's first home: the floor above Mrs. Goeppinger's Confectionary at Twenty-Second and Post Office Streets. Other sites proved no more permanent as the school regularly changed location over the next few years. Equipment shortages were another deficiency.[29] In an address given years later to the University of Texas Medical Department, James Fannin Young (J. F. Y.) Paine reported class visuals consisted of "one disarticulated skeleton, three large anatomical maps, and one obstetrical manikin" with the later addition of a "few models of the eye and ear." Bodies were needed for dissection. However, Texas state laws of the period required that all corpses must be buried. The solution? The bodies were exhumed. "The rigid exactions of the law had to be complied with," explained Paine, "and to evade its penalties the dead bodies generally underwent the formality of internment. These subjects were subsequently resurrected by the students, the ghoulish forays being undertaken after midnight in the dark of the moon and hair-raising experiences were sometimes associated with these gruesome missions."[30]

Neither location issues nor the dearth of teaching aids discouraged the energetic and ardent members of the Galveston Medical College faculty. They provided students with a full course of lectures on anatomy, chemistry, obstetrics, therapeutics, and physiology, among other subjects. Dowell also leased the Galveston City Hospital, where undergraduates could practice patient care in the overcrowded facility.[31] However, by the early 1870s, Soule University faced overwhelming odds as the school became immersed in red ink. Dowell appealed to the legislature on behalf of the college but came up short. Under the strain, Texas Methodists shifted their financial support to the recently established Southwestern University in Georgetown. Abandoned in Texas, Soule University officials closed the Chappell Hill and Galveston Medical College campuses and relocated to Louisiana.[32]

Dowell remained undaunted by Soule's departure. Rather than surrender his vision for a medical department in Galveston, the pragmatic physician simply changed course. As Soule's prospects faded, Dowell cut ties with the university and reorganized. Armed with a charter for a hospi-

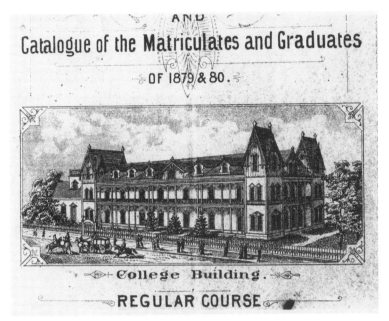

Galveston Medical College and Hospital. Advertisement published in the Galveston City Directory, 1878–1879. *Courtesy Rosenberg Library.*

tal granted by the state legislature in May 1871, Dowell, along with fellow physician J. M. Callaway, established the Texas Medical College and Hospital (TMCH). The new school continued the high academic standards of the Galveston Medical College. Candidates for professorships underwent a rigorous examination process. Students pursued a demanding curriculum of courses often taught within Dowell's stately residence on Avenue L between Twenty-First and Twenty-Second Streets. Those who persevered received a Latin-inscribed diploma upon graduation.[33]

The primary boon for the college involved the newly chartered hospital. Under legislative grant, county courts in Texas now had a respectable venue to send their indigent sick at a maximum cost of one dollar per day. The hospital admitted many patients. For instance, in 1872, the Galveston County Commissioners allocated $1,799.75 to the medical college for indigent care. Dowell, his fellow faculty members, and students of the medical college all benefited. The more indigent patients that were sent to the hospital, the greater the opportunities for clinical care and teaching. Yet, overall local and state support for the school remained deficient. Few students attended TMCH compared to those from Texas who chose to study medicine elsewhere. The hospital was insufficient as a school building, and as the 1870s progressed, state funding for the indigent seriously dwindled. The times called for a critical change.[34]

Ashbel Smith had not been idle during the years surrounding Dowell's spirited efforts to promote medical education in Texas. In the forty years since he labored over the bedsides of yellow fever patients, Smith successfully established the first hospital in Houston, published medical articles and treatises, and aided in organizing the Harris County Medical Society and the Texas Medical Association. As the doyen of the state's physicians, Smith also presided over the Texas Medical College and Hospital examining board. These achievements and many others were products of Smith's characteristic talent, determination, and chutzpah. In contrast to the imposing six-foot-tall Greensville Dowell, Smith was a diminutive man who stood little over five feet and weighed approximately 115 pounds. Those who underestimated Smith did so at their peril. The tiny physician-statesman possessed a temper that "bellowed fire" when crossed, and rarely was he known to back down in an argument. Smith displayed this aspect of his personality more than once during his three-term service in the state legislature (1855, 1866, 1879). In one instance, a fellow legislator dangled a rubber spider over Smith's ear as he dozed during a member's speech. Irritated over being the butt of a practical joke, Smith chased the perpetrator down the aisle of the House of Representatives and kicked him out the door. "Mr. Speaker," Smith reportedly remarked, "that is a practical demonstration of your governor's pay-as-you-go policy."[35]

Characteristic hotheadedness aside, Smith effectively utilized his political powers as an ardent supporter of education. A tireless champion of public education for all, including women and African Americans, Smith organized the Philosophical Society of Texas and helped establish the Stuart Female Seminary in Austin (1876–99) and Prairie View A&M University (1876). Such triumphs brought great satisfaction to the aging Smith; yet one dream remained unfulfilled. It echoed a desire expressed by Mirabeau Lamar decades before: the establishment of a state university and, with it, a first-class medical branch.[36]

Smith got his wish during the spring of 1881. On April 1, Governor Oran M. Roberts appointed Smith to the first board of regents of the University of Texas, and he was elected president of the board during its first meeting. Yet, before plans for a state university and medical school could truly get underway, a primary question needed to be resolved. Where would each institution be located? Would they share the same site, or would they be separate? The state legislature authorized Texans to answer those questions by referendum. Leading up to the election, voters overwhelmingly supported Austin as the site for the main university. The question over where to locate the University of Texas Medical Department involved considerably more debate. Civic leaders and physicians throughout Texas, especially those in Houston, Galveston, Austin, and Tyler, coveted the commerce and prestige a medical school would bring to their communities. Many influential Texans, including Ashbel Smith, supported Galveston for its size, wealth, and distinct medical culture found nowhere else in the state. Others disagreed. Austin advocates in particular argued against "dismembering" the university. How, they asked, could the university's regents adequately oversee two campuses located miles apart in a frontier, rural state? More importantly, they pointed out, the Island had a miserable reputation for hurricanes, yellow fever outbreaks, and other coastal maladies, not to mention the many diseases brought by way of immigrant ships. Indeed it did, admitted Ashbel Smith. Yet, he argued, modern medical students required practical as well as theoretical experience. Galveston, urged Smith, was the perfect location for a medical school because it possessed the greatest number of diseases for students to study. The people of Texas agreed. On September 6, 1881, Austin was chosen as the location for the main university and Galveston for the medical school. Anticipating a new and state-supported medical school in town, the Texas Medical College closed shortly afterward.[37]

Few Texans expected the procrastination that followed. Despite local enthusiasm and support, it took nearly a decade for the new University of Texas Medical Department to open its doors. The reasons behind the delay included an initial lack of state funding, a prolonged planning process, complications with purchasing the proper site, and ultimately architectural changes to the college building. In the meantime, the Texas Medical College reopened to fill the gap until the medical department was firmly on its feet. Upon his death in 1884, wealthy Galveston merchant John Sealy bequeathed $50,000 for a "charitable purpose." Sealy's widow, Rebecca, and his brother, George, allocated the money to construct the John Sealy Hospital. By 1887 plans for the medical department were on a roll. Led by Galveston millionaire Walter Gresham, then chairman of the House Finance Committee, the state legislature allotted $125,000 to the University of Texas, including $50,000 to construct the medical school. The combined generosity of both city and state enabled the purchase of land on the east end of Galveston Island to build the school.[38]

A premier school for nurses was also on the rise in Galveston. Up to this point, with the exception of nuns, unskilled male attendants were the chief administrators of nursing care in Texas hospitals. The outcome was often less than satisfactory. During the general debate over the location of the medical department, A. R. Kilpatrick, president of the Texas Medical Association, denounced traditional nursing practices. "Some nurses are nuisances," Kilpatrick proclaimed, "and drink up all the wine and stimu-

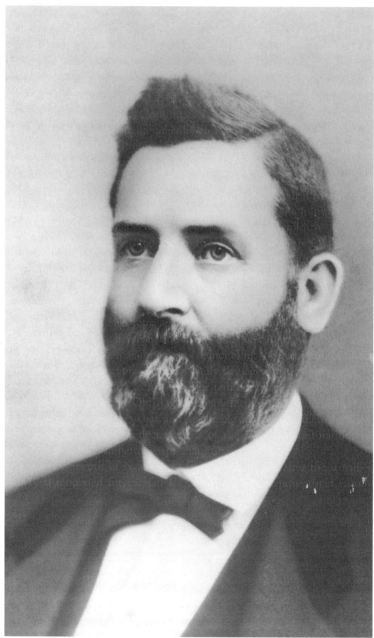

John Sealy I (1822–84). The terms of Sealy's will enabled the establishment of the John Sealy Hospital in 1890 and expedited the opening of the Medical Department in 1891. *Courtesy Blocker History of Medicine Collections, Moody Medical Library.*

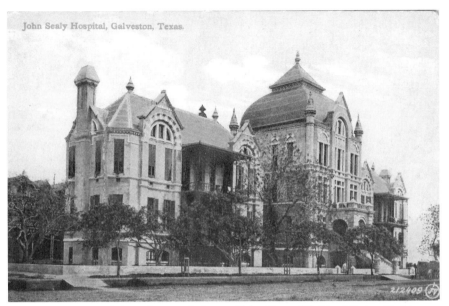

Postcard image of John Sealy Hospital. *Courtesy Blocker History of Medicine Collections, Moody Medical Library.*

lants furnished for the sick."[39] A few years later, Kilpatrick's colleague, A. P. Brown, proposed a solution. In 1884 Brown recommended the establishment of a training school for nurses that would operate in conjunction with the new medical department. In Brown's view, skilled nursing was critical to patient outcome. "Judicious nursing by trained hands," he noted, "often determines the result of a disease."[40] Yet, reform was slow in coming. Despite the opinions of professionals like Kilpatrick and Brown, most nineteenth-century physicians in Texas and throughout the South preferred the status quo to having young white women with no special training working in hospitals.

It took the accidental injury of a little girl and a resolute group of Galveston women to stimulate nursing reform in Texas. In 1889 young Ella Goldthwaite, a member of the prominent Sealy family, accidentally fell and broke her hip. The family sent the child to a specialist in New York. Little Ella returned to the Island several weeks later under the care of Dorthea Fick, a graduate of the Mount Sinai School of Nursing. Unfortunately, Ella died after a lengthy illness in January 1890. By that time, however, the efficiency of Fick's nursing skills had impressed many prominent citizens in Galveston. As a result, a group of influential, reform-minded women in Galveston created the Lady Board of Manag-

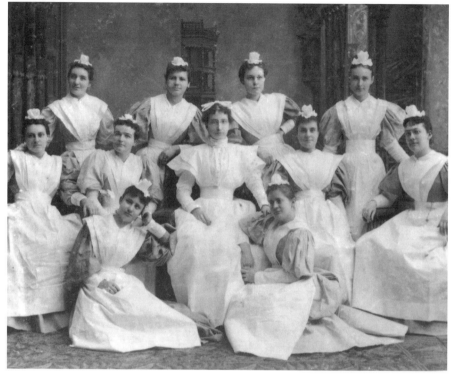

Junior Class, John Sealy Traing School for Nurses (1895). *Courtesy Blocker History of Medicine Collections, Moody Medical Library.*

ers to spearhead a training school for nurses. It was an uphill climb. With Ella Goldthwaite's mother as president, the board battled the hostility of traditionalists through argument, threats to boycott the services of older physicians in favor of younger ones, and a lucrative fundraising campaign. Through the unflagging efforts of this group of women, the John Sealy Training School for Nurses, the first nursing school in Texas, opened on March 10, 1890, with a freshman class of eighteen young women.[41]

In the midst of preparations for the nursing school, the University of Texas Board of Regents turned its attention towards faculty recruitment for the new medical department. The board created eight distinct faculty chairs and advertised these positions in American and European medical journals. Resisting convention, the regents chose an eclectic mix of energetic, idealistic, and talented physicians to fill the positions. Four of the doctors—all TMCH professors—hailed from Galveston, two from other cities in Texas, one from Philadelphia, and two from Great Britain.

The highly esteemed and gracious J. F. Y. Paine, professor of gynecology and obstetrics, served as the medical department dean. William Keiller and James Thompson of Great Britain brought the best of Old World medical traditions in anatomy and surgery. Other physician-professors included Allen J. Smith, pathology; Albert G. Clopton, physiology and hygiene; Galveston native Edward Randall, therapeutics and materia medica; Hamilton Atchinson West, medicine; and Seth Mabry Morris, chemistry. The original faculty was a young group. Only two were past middle age. The youngest member, Texan Seth Mabry Morris, was the only one to earn his undergraduate degree at the University of Texas.[42] The superintendent of the John Sealy Training School for Nurses, Hanna Kindbom, joined the medical faculty as Clinical Instructor of Nursing. Kindbom's commission was a significant step forward in nursing education, as it was the first time a nurse received a professional appointment in an academic institution.[43] Throughout their careers at the University of Texas Medical Department, each of these designated professors worked daily under a common mission: to endow their students with a first-rate medical education.

By 1891 many elements were in place for a university-based medical school. A fully operating hospital, a supply of trained nurses, and an illustrious faculty were at the ready. All the Medical Department needed now was a building.

Chapter 2

THE TALENTED MR. CLAYTON

Few, if any, architects shaped the physical characteristics of an American city more than Nicholas Joseph Clayton influenced Galveston. With an almost overwhelming talent and energy, Clayton designed and built many of the major public, commercial, and residential buildings on the Island, most of them built between 1874 and 1902. From breathtakingly ornate churches to charming gingerbread cottages, each structure was a work of art.

A premier masterpiece—considered to be one of Clayton's proudest achievements—was a magnificent edifice designed to house the University of Texas Medical Department. Constructed of red pressed brick and ruddy Texas granite, it has acquired many names: "the Medical Department building," "the main building," and "the red building." In 1949 the structure was officially designated the Ashbel Smith Building, in honor of the renowned physician. Through the years, however, one label, fondly bestowed by the school's early students and faculty has surpassed all others in popularity, "Old Red."

Nicholas Clayton had been acquainted with challenges from an early age. Born on November 1, 1840, to parents Nicholas Joseph Clayton Sr. (1797–1841) and Margaret O'Mahoney Clayton (1815–1910), young Nicholas spent his early years in the impoverished village of Cloyne, County Cork, Ireland. Despite their poverty, residents of Cloyne were proud of two outstanding features of their community. The village centerpiece was the ancient Cathedral of St. Colman (c. 1250), widely recognized, especially in the eighteenth century, for its exceptional liturgical music. The church housed an active parish of which the Claytons were a part. The massive granaries of Cloyne, the employer of Nicholas Clayton Sr. and many others, were another source of pride. However, trouble began for the Clayton family shortly after Nicholas's birth. In 1841 the elder Nicholas J. Clayton passed away, leaving his wife and young son to confront an oncoming disaster on their own. Beginning in 1845, a terrible rot attacked the potato crop, the keystone staple of Ireland. Over the next seven years, the potato famine decimated the Irish countryside. More than one million peasants succumbed to disease and hunger, their starved bodies often found along roadsides, some with grass still in their mouths. As many as two million desperate Irish fled the misery of their homeland. Many flooded onto ships offering cheap fares across the Atlantic to Canada and the United States. Thousands more died at sea in the overcrowded holds of these "coffin ships." In 1847 alone, 40,000 Irish perished at sea from dysentery, typhus, and malnutrition. Those who survived the passage often found themselves pushed into the dreary, disease-ridden slums of Boston, Philadelphia, and New York.[1]

With seven-year-old Nicholas in tow, Margaret boarded a steamer bound for America in May of 1848. They were more fortunate than many of their countrymen. Not only did mother and son survive the voyage, but Margaret possessed the financial resources necessary to avoid the abject circumstances of many newly arrived Irish. After landing in Boston, they journeyed to Cincinnati, Ohio, the hometown of her sister and brother-in-law, Mary and Daniel Crowley. Daniel Crowley's relationship with Nicholas was the closest the young man would ever have to a father-son experience. From all accounts, the remainder of Clayton's childhood was unexceptional. He attended Roman Catholic parochial schools and graduated in 1858. Crowley made his living from various building trades that eventually exposed Nicholas to the world of architecture and construction. Military records indicate Clayton worked as a plasterer in his late teens and sold his services to builders in New Orleans, Memphis, Louisville, and St. Louis.[2]

Clayton's fledgling career was soon disrupted by the Civil War. On November 18, 1862, Clayton joined the United States Navy at St. Louis. He was promoted to yeoman on December 30, 1863, and served in that rank until the end of hostilities in 1865. Clayton witnessed significant action during his naval tenure. He was first assigned to the USS *Juliet*, a gunboat that is thought to have participated in the crucial Union victory at Vicksburg (April–July 1863) where Union forces, under the command of Ulysses S. Grant, overwhelmed the Rebel stronghold on the Mississippi River and cut the Confederacy in two. The following spring, hostile fire near Alexandria, Louisiana, sent the *Juliet* limping back to port. On May 14, 1864, yeoman Clayton was transferred to another gunboat, the USS *Hastings*, for the remainder of the war. Clayton's service on both vessels provided him a deck-side view of the American Midwest. Between late 1862 and 1865, the *Juliet* and *Hastings* patrolled the waters of the Ohio, Tennessee, Cumberland, Mississippi, White, Red, and Yazoo Rivers. During the summer of 1865, Clayton disembarked for a final time. He was discharged on June 16 in Cairo, Illinois.[3]

Clayton quickly resumed his career after the war. By 1866 he was back in Cincinnati, eager to expand his skills as an artisan. Between 1866 and 1871, Clayton's name appeared in three editions of the Cincinnati City Directory. His talents broadened with each entry. He was listed as a marble carver in the 1866 edition, a stone carver in 1870, and an architectural draftsman in 1871. In *Clayton's Galveston*, architectural historians Barrie Scardino and Drexel Turner observed that the launching of Clayton's professional career coincided with a pivotal era in the history of American design. It was a time, they wrote, when "new money and new technology were united, improbably, with widespread Romanticism and a taste for the exotic and the picturesque."[4] The newly rich conspicuously displayed their wealth through a variety of High Victorian styles: Italianate, French Second Empire, Gothic, Romanesque, and Queen Anne. Residential and public buildings showcased turreted towers, picturesque massing, mansard roofs, granite archways, and decorative glass. Clayton became acquainted with these trends early in his training. His comprehension increased under the tutelage of Mathias Baldwin, co-owner of the Memphis architectural firm Jones & Baldwin.[5] By the early 1870s, Clayton had a firm grasp of building formulas, proportional composition schemes, and the elements of architectural detail. The only thing he lacked was on-the-job experience.

That opportunity presented itself with a trip to Galveston. In April of 1872, Jones & Baldwin sent Clayton to the island city as the supervising architect for the second Tremont Hotel (the first hotel, built in 1837, burned down during the Civil War) and the First Presbyterian Church. Contemporary accounts described the firm's Norman-style design for the church, with its formal elegance and 190-foot spire, as the most magnificent in Galveston since the Civil War. For Clayton, the assignment offered numerous lessons in the practical side of his profession: how to organize an on-site office, woo clients, and prepare drawings for presentations and construction blueprints. He had ample chance to learn. Dependent upon parish proceeds, occasionally supplied solely from ice cream socials, construction on the First Presbyterian Church took four years to complete (1872–76). Clayton took advantage of the wait by developing his own business. By 1874 Clayton mastered the professional ropes enough to establish his own firm with the blessing of Jones & Baldwin.[6]

It was a timely move. During these years, Galveston was rapidly becoming the cultural and professional capital of Texas, with the largest banks and commercial enterprises in the state. Tremendous fortunes were in the making, and construction projects sprang up throughout the city. Up to this point, Galveston had lacked a professional architect. Clayton was ideally suited to fill the gap. In 1874 Clayton listed himself as "architect" in the Galveston City Directory and began advertising in local newspapers.

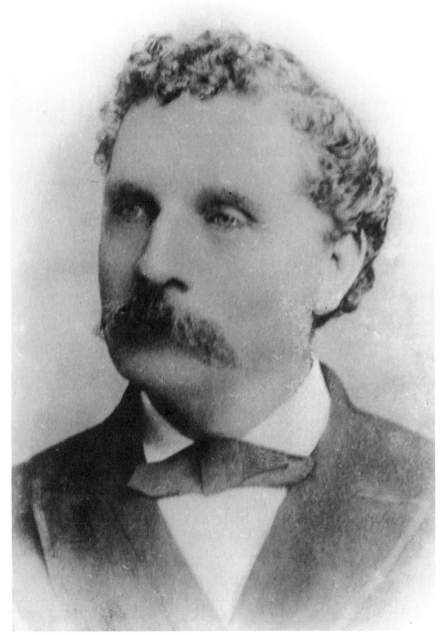

Nicholas J. Clayton (1840–1916). *Courtesy Rosenberg Library.*

One ad published in the *Galveston Daily News* claimed Clayton the "Earliest Established Professional Architect in the State." Clayton's architectural talents were perfectly suited to the flamboyant tastes of Galveston's elite. His work embraced the eclecticism of High Victorian style, heavy on ornamental detail. Yet, Clayton's creative application of contrasting colors and textures, rich ornamentation, and proportional order distinguished his architectural style from that of other Texas architects. He was prolific as well. Between 1874 and 1902, Clayton built an astounding number of structures—totaling over 225—in Galveston alone. His first recorded independent commission, the Island City Savings Bank, was followed by a variety of projects: financial institutions and other businesses, hospitals, churches, schools, grand homes, and intimate cottages. His reputation quickly spread beyond Galveston. Within the whole of his career, Clayton designed, built, or remodeled buildings in sixteen other Texas cities, four southern states, and Mexico.[7]

Called "N. J." by his friends, Nicholas Clayton's persona contrasted sharply with that of his brusque, gem-bridled clients. He was quiet and reserved with a soft sense of humor. Even at the zenith of his career, Clayton's name rarely appeared in the society or community columns of local Galveston newspapers. He possessed an average height—five feet, ten inches—and sported an athletic build that he kept in condition through long daily walks and regular dips in Galveston Bay. He had dark brown curly hair, clear, blue eyes, and a ruddy complexion. Clayton dressed fastidiously, taking great pride in his appearance throughout his life. Each workday found him in an immaculately tailored suit and bow tie even when inspecting construction sites. In his later years, the architect bore a striking resemblance to Mark Twain as he kept his full, gray hair long, and complemented his suits with a soft black silk four-in-hand. Throughout his life, Clayton remained a devout Catholic and attended mass daily. For many years, he devoted his free time to entertaining children at St. Mary's Orphanage, surprising them with gifts and managing the annual New Year's Eve fireworks display.[8]

Perhaps his reserve kept Clayton a bachelor far longer than most men. Around 1873, Clayton brought his mother, Margaret Clayton, from Cincinnati to live with him. Mother and son lived together in a small raised cottage at Avenue L and Thirty-Sixth Street for twenty years. Clayton finally broke his bachelorhood at age fifty-one. On July 6, 1892, Clayton married twenty-six-year-old Mary Lorena Ducie (1865–1944) in St. Mary's Cathedral. Even then, his choice of bride reflected a hesitancy to venture out of an immediate social circle. Mary Lorena was the daughter of Confederate Major Daniel W. Ducie, an English artisan-decorator and close collaborator on several construction projects, including the elaborate four-storied Bishop's Palace. After a monthlong honeymoon to Monterrey, Mexico, the couple set up housekeeping in a house located on the corner of Thirty-Fifth Street and Avenue L. In this residence, they raised a thriving family of five children: Daniel Louis (1893–1924), Nicholas Joseph Jr. (1895–1974), Mary Margaret (1897–1986), Theresa Rose (1898–1924), and John Charles (1902–86). Nicholas and Mary remained devoted to each other for over twenty-five years. The family owned the home on Thirty-Fifth and Avenue L until the passing of Mary Clayton in 1944.[9]

Although Clayton often worked independently, he engaged in two partnerships during the course of his career. In 1877 he partnered with fellow Irishman Michael L. Lynch, a civil engineer. The firm Clayton & Lynch lasted until 1881; sometime afterward, Lynch relocated to Fort Worth. The duo is noted for designing a series of commercial buildings along the Strand, including Ball, Hutchings and Company; Wallis, Landes and Company; Schneider and Company; and Marx and Kempner. The other partnership included Patrick Rabbit Jr., a young Irishman who joined Clayton & Lynch as a trainee. In 1890 the senior architect made Rabbit a partner and formed N. J. Clayton and Company with offices located in the T. J. League Building at 2307 Strand.

When American architects began to organize professionally in the mid-1870s, Clayton threw his support behind many societies and associations on the ground floor. In 1886 he became one of twenty-one charter members of the Association of Texas Architects, a state chapter of the Western Association of Architects (WAA). He became a fellow of the American Institute of Architects (AIA) when it absorbed the WAA in 1889. Clayton served as vice president of the Southern Chapter of AIA from 1895–96. In addition to professional affiliations, Clayton participated in fraternal organizations and civic societies. These included the Catholic Knights of America, the Knights of Columbus, the Ancient Order of Hibernians, and the Garten Verein.[10]

Clayton assumed an enormous workload during most of his career. The height of commissions occurred in the years following the Galveston fire of 1885 that devastated over forty blocks in the city's east end. Clayton's eclectic talents and good taste were widely sought by patrons rebuilding the area. An office diary from 1887 shows Clayton overseeing sixty-four projects during this period.[11] Effective management of such a load required incredible self-discipline, strong management skills, and a heavy dose of genius, all characteristics the architect possessed. He normally worked at an intense pace: on average fifty-five hours per week, taking off only on Sundays. He was a perfectionist, whose architectural plans were meticulously organized and left nothing to chance. Upon receipt of a contract, Clayton's office produced precise pen-and-ink drawings and charts, specified to chosen materials. Except for structures of extraordinary size and scale, the process between design and construction took twelve months on average to complete. There were times when the architect produced a masterpiece in extremely short order. According to Clayton's wife, Mary Lorena, the architect completed the unique plans for the Garten Verein in a single night.[12] Concentration was vital, however. Having grown up next door to the Clayton home, John McGivney remembered watching the architect at work. "We were allowed to stand as close as we wished to watch him," he recalled, "just so long as we did not joggle his arm or talk above a whisper."[13]

Clayton rarely spent time in the office. In addition to providing designs for buildings, Clayton assumed the role of general contractor as well. He insisted upon personally supervising each project under construction down to the inspection of all work and materials. He was fair-minded in his business dealings but tough with substandard operations of any kind. Clayton's office journal reveals episodes where he terminated contractors and contacted a lumberyard to pick up an inferior product it had sent out previously.[14]

As Galveston's premier architect and builder, Clayton never lacked for skilled help. He had his pick from one of the finest corps of craftsmen ever assembled in Texas: carpenter artists, masons, and stone carvers—many of them immigrants from Western Europe. They included Denny Devlin, Clayton's favorite master brick mason; John Stephenson, Dick Koeppe, and Billy Cohea, carpenters; and John O'Brien, stone mason. Clayton placed a great premium on structural interiors and often utilized the decorating and painting skills of his father-in-law, Daniel Ducie. Other relatives assisted as well. Brother-in-law William Ducie often did his graining work. Clayton's uncle Daniel Crowley, who moved from Cincinnati to Houston in the 1870s, administered the skillful modeling and embellishment of Eaton Chapel of Trinity Episcopal in 1878–79. Clayton also took full advantage of the late-nineteenth-century improvements in communication and transportation to shop swiftly and lavishly. Telegraph wires, the mails, shipping lanes, and rails enabled Clayton to continuously send and receive samples of building materials. He acquired cut marble from Italy and Africa; onyx and mahogany from Mexico; and beautiful woods of cherry, maple, and ash from Vermont. Bricks and tiles manufactured in England, Belgium, and Philadelphia arrived on ships in exchange for cotton. Clayton enjoyed choice selections of limestone and pink granite dug from Texas quarries and lacy cast-iron trim transported from New Orleans or produced by Galveston's own foundries.[15]

For more than three decades, Nicholas Clayton created architectural

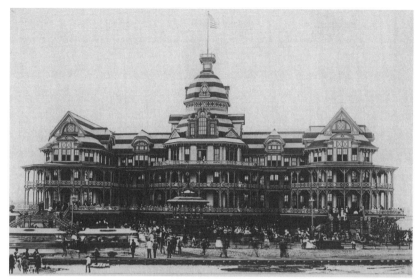

The Beach Hotel (1882). Designed by Nicholas Clayton, the Beach Hotel opened for visitors on July 4, 1883. Hotel amenities included a gentleman's parlor, saloon, reading room and menagerie of exotic animals. The ornate, wooden structure was destroyed by fire in 1898. *Courtesy Rosenberg Library.*

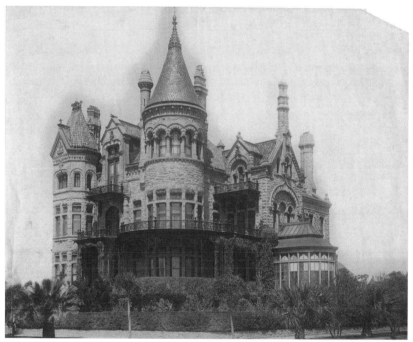

Walter Gresham Home, known as the "Bishop's Palace" (1892). Built of stone and steel, this Clayton-designed structure is one of Galveston's most outstanding historic buildings. *Courtesy Rosenberg Library.*

legacies in Galveston that still remain a source of pride and distinction. Fif-teen edifices on the Strand are credited to Clayton, including the Kauffman & Runge (now Stewart Title) Building (220 Twenty-Second Street), the Romanesque-arched Galveston News Building (2108 Mechanic Street), and the cast-iron columned W. L. Moody Building (2202–2206 Strand). Each stone and brick structure projects a summary statement of power through conspicuous columns, carved scrolls, elaborate cornices, and other ornamental expressions. Clayton designed picturesque wooden pleasure palaces, including the gabled Galveston Electric Pavilion (1881–83), the first building in Texas with electric lighting, and the charming, ginger-bread-latticed Garten Verein (2704 Avenue O). Most striking of all was the three-story, three-pavilioned Beach Hotel (1883–98). Rising up 18 feet out of the sand, the hotel was enormous: 245 feet in length with 18-foot-wide verandas wrapped around the front and sides of the building. Perhaps the structure's most captivating feature was the paint scheme. The main body of the building, painted mauve with golden green accents, was topped with a red-and-white-striped roof. The dome was finished in a variety of colors, and the ridges attached to the roofs of the east and west pavilions were adorned with iron cresting painted bronze and gold. Yet, Clayton's work was not solely reserved for the public sphere. Evidence of his hand can be found along many of the Island's residential streets, from graceful, intimate cottages to lavish three-storied mansions complete with columns, turrets, spires, and intricate ironwork. The grandest of Clayton's residential com-missions is the Walter Gresham home, commonly known as the "Bishop's Palace." Located at 1402 Broadway, the three-story home epitomized Clay-ton's architectural inventiveness and eye for superb craftsmanship.[16]

Ecclesiastical design was Clayton's greatest passion. Although he enjoyed creating all types of buildings, the deeply religious architect adored churches. His affinity for them was based not only as temples of faith, but sanctuaries in a harsh world. The roots of Clayton's reverence for church design most likely originated during his childhood when the village cathedral at Cloyne provided comfort from his famine-infested environment. Like most artists, Clayton doodled constantly, whether in meetings, in the midst of casual conversations, or during a quiet moment. Surviving sketches reveal an artist enamored with church altars, windows, steeples, and sacred ornamentation. An early example of Clayton's affec-tion for churches occurred the very first day he arrived in Galveston. On that December day in 1872, the newcomer alighted from the Galveston railroad station and proceeded to St. Mary's Cathedral to attend mass. As he passed by a shop window on Market Street, he stopped to admire two Seth Thomas clocks and a bisque Madonna and child. On a whim, Clayton purchased the items and ordered them sent around the corner to

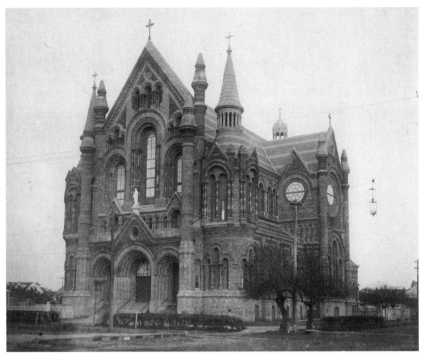

Sacred Heart Catholic Church, Galveston (demolished 1900). *Courtesy Rosenberg Library.*

his temporary quarters at the old Washington Hotel on Twenty-First and Mechanic. Clayton continued on to the mass and then lingered afterwards in order to introduce himself to Bishop Claude Dubuis. The two men developed a warm relationship. Over time, the young architect persuaded Dubois to allow him to render a few architectural changes to St. Mary's, including the addition of a central tower to balance the two towers in front of the basilica. The project began in 1875, shortly after a hurricane swept across the Island, destroying portions of the Texas Gulf Coast. Although Galveston survived the storm, Clayton built the tower and as a symbolic gesture crowned the structure with an eighteen-foot statue of Mary, Star of the Sea, positioned to look out over the Island and protect it. This statue, according to local legend, acts as Galveston's protectress and has remained in place through all subsequent storms.[17]

When choosing an architect for their projects, many church officials preferred Clayton's work over others. He not only possessed a deep and impressive understanding of ecclesiastical design principles, but Clayton's ardent Catholicism enabled him to give respect and reverence to many faiths. As a result, his church commissions were multi-denominational.

The architect designed, built, added to, or remodeled many sanctuaries, including St. Patrick's Catholic Church (1013–1027 Thirty-Fourth Street), St. Mary's Cathedral (2011 Church Street), Sacred Heart Catholic Church (1302 Broadway), Eaton Memorial Chapel of Trinity Episcopal (721 Twenty-Second Street), Temple B'Nai Israel (816 Twenty-Second Street), and Grace Episcopal Church (3612 Avenue L).[18] All structures exhibit Clayton's handsome lines, model proportion, and vigorous detail. The architect undoubtedly enjoyed the satisfaction of not only viewing these houses of worship throughout the city, but even from his home. His daughter Mary remembered, "Papa used to be able to look out one door of our home on 35th and see St. Patrick's Church and out the other door see the (Grace) Episcopal Church, both buildings he had designed."[19]

Galveston was not the only recipient of Clayton's talents. As his reputation spread, Clayton traveled extensively, creating public buildings, churches, houses, and schools in many towns and cities throughout Texas. These include the R. E. Stafford Bank and Opera House (1886–87) in Columbus; the Annunciation Church (1884–1889) and Incarnate Word Academy (1905) in Houston; Sacred Heart Church (1890–1903) in Palestine; and the Sacred Heart Cathedral (1896–1902) in Dallas. Clayton's love of churches also extended outside of Texas. Project destinations included New Orleans, New Iberia, Monroe, and Baton Rouge, Louisiana; Mobile, Alabama; Tampa, Florida; and Matehuala, San Luis Potosí, Mexico.[20]

Like other Americans, nineteenth-century Texans placed high importance upon the architectural elegance of their academic institutions. From the university to the elementary level, school buildings in Texas were considered expressions of community dignity and purpose. Each structure was built to reflect the progressive cultivation of higher learning and self-improvement. Large, wealthy communities constructed school buildings that abounded in classical and medieval architectural elements. Multiple stories, large classrooms, ample use of cupolas, towers, and elaborate brickwork suggested a strong intellectual character and vision for a better future. Smaller communities with fewer funds often adopted a straightforward, less ornamental design for their school buildings. All communities constructed their school buildings to convey an enlightened respect for higher learning. In 1883 University of Texas (UT) Board of Regents President Ashbel Smith championed these sentiments on the university level. At the groundbreaking ceremonies of the UT Main Building Smith noted, "A university as a temple of knowledge is preeminently entitled to buildings of solid structure and graceful architecture with convenient rooms." Austin architect F. E. Ruffini designed the Main Building in the High Victorian Gothic style. The four-story building was constructed of pressed brick and cut stone. Cast-iron cornices and porticoes embellished

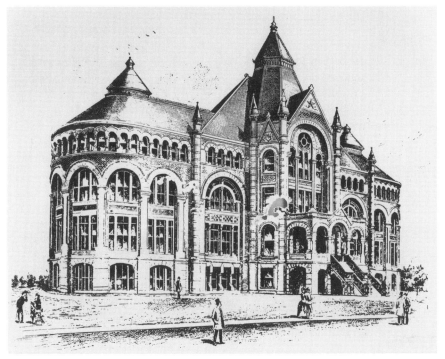

Architectural rendering of Old Red that appeared in the first Medical Department Catalogue (1891–92). *Courtesy Blocker History of Medicine Collections, Moody Medical Library.*

the exterior, while exposed metalwork added interior interest. Nicholas Clayton incorporated the picturesque Victorian Gothic in his design of another Austin academic institution, St. Edwards College (1888–89, 1903). Located on an imposing site approximately three miles from the state capitol, the school building is an imposing structure characterized by refined, raised brickwork, pointed arches, and an angular silhouette. However, when it came time to design a medical school, Clayton had a different vision in mind.[21]

In 1888 the University of Texas finally received the nod to begin constructing a medical school. The state legislature allocated $50,000 to UT for the purpose. With funds in place, the UT Board of Regents issued a call for proposals from architects. The search eventually narrowed to four competitors: Nicholas J. Clayton, W. J. Roystone, Thomas J. Wood, and Alfred Muller. As the creator of the neighboring Renaissance-style John Sealy Hospital, Clayton had an edge over his competitors. The regents selected his plans in early September 1888. However, project delays ensued almost immediately. The regents realized that the previously purchased block 668 was not large enough for both John Sealy Hospital and the new medical school building. In search of additional territory, regent T. C. Thompson of Galveston began bargaining with local landowners. After more than a year, Thompson succeeded in acquiring lots on block 669 that became the site for Old Red. The Texas Legislature agreed to provide $25,000 for the purchase if the city of Galveston would donate matching funds for the entire construction project. A deal was cut, and Clayton revised his original plans to accommodate the new space.[22]

Before he drew up the final plans for the school, Clayton wanted to ensure he had thoroughly researched the project. He proposed a fact-finding tour of the North and East to acquire "the most modern . . . ideas as to the construction and equipment of medical colleges." The UT regents granted Clayton's request and allocated $150 for the trip. During his tour, Clayton visited a number of noteworthy medical schools, including Johns Hopkins, the University of Pennsylvania, the College of Physicians and Surgeons in New York, and Harvard University. At each stop, Clayton took extensive notes as he researched the "general design arrangement and construction of the . . . scientific departments and their subdivisions, the laboratory, dissecting room and attending offices, furnishings and administrative requisites." In the midst of his tour, Clayton realized that very few American medical schools had the advantage of having both their medical school building and companion hospital on the same campus. Clayton made critical alterations to his plans upon his return to Galveston. His changes included the installation of skylights in the amphitheaters and over the tables for anatomy and chemistry demonstrations, extra storage space for chemical and anatomical specimens, and increased ventilation in classrooms and laboratories.[23]

Construction on the medical department building commenced in the fall of 1889. In October the general construction contract for $69,000 was awarded to August Baumbach, a Houston builder. The *Galveston Daily News* noted Baumbach possessed a statewide reputation "as an able and trustworthy contractor, and one who operates on a large scale." Workers began building Old Red in November. Less than two months later, the adjoining John Sealy Hospital opened on January 10, 1890. During the first three weeks of operation, the institution serviced ninety inpatients and twenty-two outpatients. However, the hospital suffered from inadequate nursing care until the John Sealy Hospital Training School for Nurses began functioning in March 1890 with student nurses who learned their skills as they dispensed care to patients. By the following autumn, doctors and nurses had successfully treated over 1,400 patients in all.[24]

By December 1890, the basic structure of Old Red was complete. But there remained a problem. The legislature had not provided funds for the

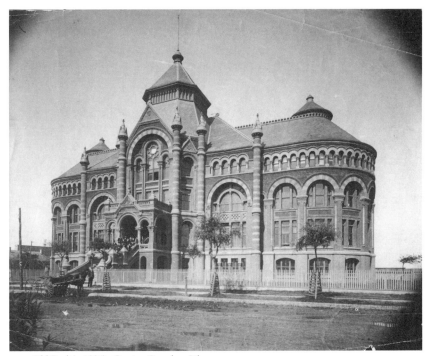

Old Red (c. 1894). *Courtesy Rosenberg Library.*

purchase of equipment and furniture for the building, not to mention faculty salaries. It would take several more months to receive adequate funding to begin operations. On October 5, 1891, the new University of Texas Medical Department building was ready to receive the first group of students.

On opening day, the public beheld one of the finest examples of Clayton's architectural genius. Commanding a beautiful view of the Gulf of Mexico on one side and the bay and shipyards on the other, Old Red is a magnificent masterpiece of red brick and limestone. The building is massive, extending three stories above an elevated, pier-supported basement and measuring two hundred by sixty-eight feet, excluding portico and other additions to the exterior. The central roof measures approximately one hundred and twenty feet in height. Clayton designed the building in the Victorian Romanesque style. Distinctive features of this architectural style include arcading, which refers to a row of arches applied to the wall for decoration; decorated bricks and terra-cotta tiles in conjunction with stone trim; round arches supported by short, polished stone columns; superficial ornamentation; and different colored and textured stone or brick for window trim. But Clayton did not stop there. In addition to these features, the architect rhythmically blended into his creation other architecturally distinct styles—Romanesque arcades, Italian Gothic gables, and Moorish pinnacles—on a massive scale, highly reminiscent of the numerous ethnic groups that mingled daily along Galveston's wharves. Immigrant masons and bricklayers used Cedar Bayou pressed brick, red Texas granite, and sandstone to construct the curved arches, pilasters, buttresses, and gallery of windows. The expertise of master brick mason Denny Devlin guaranteed an elaborate structural façade with layered arches, corbels, diagonal brick patterning, and angled bond. Polished columns of red Texas granite adorn the entrance with encaustic tiles placed on the front porticoes. The original blue and green tiled roof (now terracotta colored) added further embellishment to the rich exterior.

The interior of Old Red was also exceptional. With an eye for functional yet elegant style, Clayton incorporated the most contemporary elements of medical institution design. The top floor contained a large, skylit dissecting room that provided ample space to house a large collection of specimens acquired from anatomical and pathological museums. The other floors contained three spacious lecture amphitheaters; laboratories for chemistry, physiology, histology, pathology, and bacteriology; a library; and offices for faculty. A broad, sweeping staircase of Texas pine and cypress connected the three floors and basement.

Throughout the designing of Old Red, Clayton always kept the uniqueness of the building site in mind. In contrast to other medical schools throughout the country, the UT Medical Department building and neighboring John Sealy Hospital were situated on a Gulf Coast peninsula. Therefore, Clayton incorporated many features specifically designed for warm, humid summers, short winters, and rapid changes in the weather. These included a hipped roof, semicircular shaped east and west wings, and vertical circulation devices in the central portion of the building. The *Galveston Daily News* described the building as "most suitable, not only on its merits of light and ventilation, but also the superior interior acoustic properties and external architectural effects." The newspaper also noted, "Such climatic necessities and requirements have been learned . . . from a long residence and an extended experience in the handling of all classes of public and private buildings in this city." Clayton had been a practicing architect in Galveston eighteen years by the time Old Red was completed. Perhaps no other structure in Clayton's repertoire better reflected his deep, physical acquaintance with his adopted home.[25]

For the rest of his life, Old Red remained a source of great pride for Nicholas Clayton. In addition to its being one of Clayton's largest and most prestigious commissions, the structure was a masterwork of academic elegance and ornamentation on a grand scale. Perhaps best of all for Clayton, the building survived the disasters that claimed many of his other works. In 1898 the lavish Beach Hotel, host to numerous dignitaries including President Benjamin Harrison, mysteriously caught fire and burned to the ground. Sick at home, Clayton watched the heartbreaking inferno from his bedroom window. Then came the hurricane of 1900. Many of Clayton's masterpieces, including the magnificent Sacred Heart Church, celebrated as the largest church in the Southwest, were either severely damaged or destroyed. The loss of so much of his life's work, accompanied by severe financial woes resulting from a lawsuit against former partner Patrick Rabbit, were staggering setbacks for the aging architect. Outwardly, Clayton remained composed and busily engaged in various projects. But his heyday had passed.[26]

Nicholas Clayton's career ended on November 22, 1916. Aged seventy-six and still in good health, Clayton was using a candle to inspect a crack in his bedroom chimney when his shirt caught fire. He managed to squelch the flames by snatching a blanket off the bed, dunking it in a pail of water, and rolling in it. Clayton still suffered serious burns over a large portion of his body. While in the process of recovering from his ordeal, Clayton contracted pneumonia and died virtually penniless on December 9, 1916. The *Galveston Daily News* had very little to say about the illustrious architect's passing. Only a brief obituary was published in commemoration. Clayton was buried at Calvary Cemetery, 2506 Sixty-Fifth Street, a burial ground he had previously mapped out. However, his family could not afford a headstone and for many years, one of Clayton's granite samples was used to mark his grave. The situation greatly saddened his wife, Mary Lorena. She often worried that a proper monument would never be erected in her husband's memory. One day, an old family friend, Rabbi Henry Cohen of Temple B'Nai Israel set Mary's mind at ease. "Oh, you don't need one, my dear Mary Lorena," Cohen said softly, and citing the epitaph of British architectural genius, Sir Christopher Wren, Cohen consoled, "If you seek his monument, look around you."[27]

Chapter 3

TIMES OF TURMOIL AND TRIUMPH

IT WAS EARLY AUTUMN in Galveston, October 5, 1891. The summer heat had lifted, and a cool, soft breeze stroked the crowd assembled in front of Nicholas Clayton's majestic red brick edifice for the opening ceremonies of the University of Texas Medical Department. Ashbel Smith had not lived to see this day. His tough body had given out five years earlier at the age of eighty-one and was interred with high civic and military honors at the Texas State Cemetery in Austin. But the passion of Smith, Greensville Dowell, and other Texas medical pioneers was ever present that morning as Dean J. F.Y. Paine, a giant of a man standing six feet four inches tall and dressed in his customary attire of Prince Albert coat, striped trousers, ascot tie, and cream-colored beaver hat, proclaimed in his opening address the goals and expectations for the new medical school. "We are in the dawn of a new era in the history of medical education in this country," declared Paine, "and our regents . . . have organized this school upon a plan that is in line with the leading medical colleges of the United States and we are here to register the solemn edict: its standards shall never trail in the dust."[1]

Emboldened by the spirits of his medical predecessors, Paine set the bar high. The University of Texas Medical Department would not only train physicians but also fundamentally contribute to the health and well-being of the entire state of Texas. At the close of Paine's stirring remarks, the vanguard of this mission—thirteen faculty members and twenty-three students—ascended the front steps of the new school, filed under the ornate portico, and into the cool interior hallway. At that moment, Old Red began to breathe and come alive.

Paine's opening day optimism concealed a great deal of distress. Far from serene, the realities of life at the Medical Department during its early years were riddled with anxiety. Natural and fiscal adversity continually befell those laboring under Old Red's roof. While Galveston in the late nineteenth century was the richest, most sophisticated city in the state—the hub of medical resources and professionalism—it was no Eden.

"Galveston in those days rose low out of the sea," pathology professor Allen J. Smith later remembered. The city streets "were deep with sand" and the alleys "disgraceful and menacing." Like many towns and cities of its day, sanitary conditions were marginal. Outdoor privies were prevalent throughout the city. Daily drinking water was collected from "dirty roofs" and unscreened cisterns.[2] Upon his arrival to Galveston, chemistry professor Seth Mabry Morris was appalled to discover the local water "was literally alive with wiggletails" and required straining through a cloth before using. Otherwise, Morris colorfully noted, "it would have been meat as well as drink."[3] Garbage and trash cluttered the streets and alleys except during the spring and summer months when fears of yellow fever encouraged municipal clean-up campaigns. Primitive transportation services posed another inconvenience. Smith recalled citizens paid to ride in "little streetcars pulled each by a single tiny mule," and, in his view, appeared content to live completely isolated by water from the mainland except for a "single railroad bridge across the bay upheld as upon stilts by wooden piling."[4]

Although the rusticity of Galveston life could be problematic for those at the medical school, money concerns posed a greater headache. State funding for the school came from general revenues. However, despite the sincere efforts by legislators to support a sustainable medical school, the appropriated funds rarely corresponded with the amount requested by the UT regents, and a compromised amount often still fell short of the need. Issues surrounding money—or the lack thereof—soon became apparent to entering faculty during the early years.[5]

Shortly after his arrival from Manchester, England, in late summer of 1891, James E. Thompson acquired a glimpse of the prospective challenges that lay ahead. The young surgery professor had eagerly answered a solicitation for new faculty members posted in the *British Medical Journal*. According to the advertisement, the new Texas medical school and adjoining hospital buildings were "fitted with all the necessary equipment for the teaching of medicine and surgery and the ancillary sciences."[6] Thompson's first tour of Old Red revealed a different picture. "Try to imagine," he later reflected, "a series of empty rooms, scantily furnished and almost void of equipment." As Thompson entered the lofty dissecting room on the top floor of Old Red, he beheld for the first time his future friend and colleague, Scottish anatomy professor William Keiller, at work surrounded by a series of tables, upon which rested several shroud-wrapped bodies. Other than the corpses, Thompson discovered the anatomy repertoire consisted of only "a few stone crocks, a skull, several *papier mache* models of the human body and special sense organs, and a set of models of the viscera." There were no skeletons, nor prepared dissections.

Moreover, Thompson learned the school lacked a library. The closest thing was located in the basement: "a huge space, with a sand floor . . . littered with journals thrown higgledy piggledy in disorderly heaps upon the floor."[7] Conditions were little better in the classroom space assigned to pathology professor Allen J. Smith. Newly arrived from Philadelphia, Smith encountered sparsely equipped laboratories thickly covered with wood chips and shavings. As a consequence, Smith later recalled, his "first laboratory work" inside Old Red "was with a broom."[8]

Such scenes as those witnessed by Thompson, Smith, and others were quickly remedied when the state legislature provided the means to purchase enough furniture, equipment, and supplies to fill many of Old Red's empty spaces. Additional generosity arrived from members of the Galveston County Medical Society, who donated several hundred medical volumes and periodicals as the basis for a school library. However, benevolence on the behalf of the medical school continued to be touch-and-go throughout the first decade. For instance, the regents requested a total of $100,000 for school "maintenance and support" covering the biennium 1891–93. They received $75,000.[9] At times nerves wore thin. "Every second [biennial] year the legislature held our very existence in the balance," James Thompson recalled. "In its most generous moods it never gave us more than a bare sustenance . . . For many years the chair of surgery had an annual appropriation of $50 and I remember, very distinctly, feeling quite wealthy when it was raised to $100."[10]

Each academic department competed for the legislative money doled out by the university regents, and some faculty members lobbied creatively for their slice of the pie. In an effort to finance a clinical laboratory for students working the wards, Professor of Medicine James W. McLaughlin established a primitive version in the basement of John Sealy Hospital. During a visit by the regents to Galveston, McLaughlin persuaded the group to visit his little laboratory. As they entered the small, sparsely equipped room, McLaughlin proceeded to speak on the advantages of modern research facilities. An impatient regent interrupted him, asking to be shown the laboratory. "Gentlemen," McLaughlin gently countered, "you are now in the Clinical Laboratory of the University, and you behold all of our splendid equipment."[11] Chemistry professor Seth Mabry Morris was even more conspicuous in his attempt to upgrade his classroom and laboratory space. During visits to the campus by legislative committee members, Morris set to work within his poorly ventilated laboratory evaporating dishes of ammonia and hydrochloric acid and stirring up hydrogen sulfide gas. The subsequent fumes almost drove the sneezing, tearing, and coughing legislators from the medical college

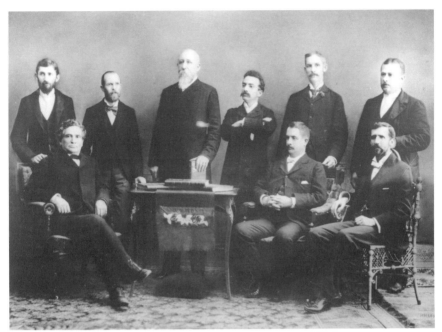

Medical Department Faculty (1895). Standing from left: Seth Mabry Morris, William Keiller, J. F. Y. Paine, Raoul Rene Cline, Edward Randall, and Allen J. Smith. Seated from left: Albert G. Clopton, Hamilton Atchinson West, and James E. Thompson. *Courtesy Blocker History of Medicine Collections, Moody Medical Library.*

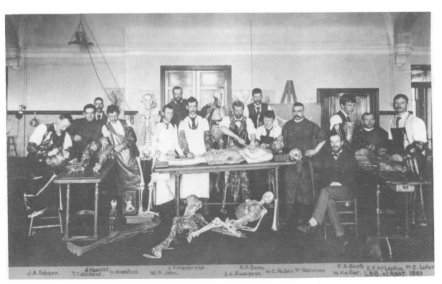

Anatomy Lab, Old Red (1891). William Keiller is seated in the foreground in striped trousers. *Courtesy Blocker History of Medicine Collections, Moody Medical Library.*

building. Despite such tactics, it took several years before Morris procured an updated laboratory for the chemistry department.[12]

As demonstrated by McLaughlin and Morris, anxieties over state funding did little to suppress the spirits of the early medical school faculty and student body. "We felt," James Thompson later asserted, "that the burden we had to carry was heavy, and that the creation of a school of medicine which would live up to the high standards of teaching to which we aspire, would require years of toil, individual sacrifice and united effort."[13] During the first ten years, Medical Department faculty members attended patients—both private and charity—in the John Sealy and St. Mary's Hospitals, prepared lectures, wrote books and journal articles, and participated in professional associations. They expected the same high level of achievement from their students. "We are no teachers of schoolboys," William Keiller counseled the student body in 1893.[14] Many early students met this challenge. In addition to maintaining a rigorous course load, they joined faculty and alumni in various professional capacities on the local, state, and national levels. They attended meetings, presented papers, and engaged in organizational politics. The magnitude of both student and faculty participation was extraordinary considering that travel in the late nineteenth century was limited to the horse and carriage, railroad, or ships.[15]

An intriguing sidelight involved the work of Professor Allen J. Smith. In addition to founding a respected pathology museum for the Medical Department, Smith engaged in a variety of research endeavors. He researched the causes and prevention of mouth infections and discovered the hookworm ova that eventually led to the establishment of hookworm disease as endemic to the southern United States. Hansen's Disease, or leprosy, was another research interest of Smith's. Experiments conducted in his laboratory implicated bedbugs as carriers of the dreaded ailment. In need of a case study, Smith hired a leper as janitor for Old Red. The arrangement ended when a bright student recognized the case and made it public.[16]

The Medical Department expanded rapidly during its first decade. In 1893, two years after Old Red opened its doors, the UT regents added the School of Pharmacy. The first professor of pharmacy, James Kennedy, succumbed to tuberculosis in 1895. For the next twenty years, Kennedy's successor, Raoul Rene Daniel Cline, fondly remembered by students for his swallow-tailed dress coat, taught pharmacy and botany. The School of Pharmacy played a viable role in the life of Old Red until 1927 when the regents moved the school to the main university in Austin. The School of Nursing also fell under the Medical Department umbrella. By the mid-1890s, the task of maintaining the John Sealy Training School for Nurses became too arduous for the Lady Board of Managers. In 1896 the UT

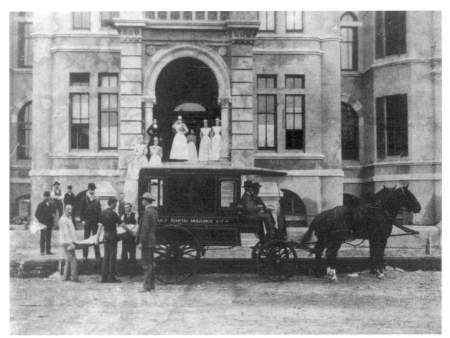

Horse-drawn ambulance in front of John Sealy Hospital (c. 1900). *Courtesy Blocker History of Medicine Collections, Moody Medical Library.*

regents relieved the board, assumed official control of the school, and changed its name to the University of Texas School of Nursing. The move was significant. For the first time in the history of the United States, a nursing school became an official unit of a university.[17]

By 1900 four primary buildings occupied the four-acre medical school campus. The focal points were Old Red and the John Sealy Hospital. Also included were the Nurses Home, a gingerbread clapboard building and University Hall, a three-story brick and terra-cotta residential facility for female medical and pharmacy.[18]

During the early years, Old Red served as the backdrop for a series of dramatic episodes that affected campus life. Two such events occurred during the 1897–98 school year. Throughout the nineteenth century, the port of Galveston not only ensured the economic health of the city, but also kept the medical school and hospitals busy. Through the port came a share of the world's diseases. Smallpox, typhoid, cholera, and pneumonia arrived on a regular basis, thus providing medical students and faculty with abundant clinical material to study. But there were drawbacks to this arrangement. Galveston was susceptible to incoming threats of infectious disease. The most dangerous of all was yellow fever. In 1867 the deadliest onslaught of "yellow jack" in Galveston claimed over 1,150 lives, or almost one-tenth of the population.[19] By the early 1900s, the scientific community had discovered the vector of yellow fever. Until then, Galveston citizens lived a precarious coexistence with the mosquito. For most of the year, recalled Seth Mabry Morris, the influx of mosquitoes was "unbearable." It was a time, Morris recollected, before windows had screens, "insect sprays were unknown," and individuals slept "under hot mosquito bars over the beds." Sitting on a neighborhood porch in early evening "meant a real fight with towels and fans."[20] For thirty years after the horrific epidemic of 1867, the vigorous enforcement of quarantine by Galveston public health officials kept yellow fever cases at a minimum. Nevertheless, in early October 1897—only days after the beginning of the medical school year—yellow fever hit the Island again.

Denial was the first response. Galveston physicians overwhelmingly maintained that dengue was the source of the local fever cases. However, as an experienced observer of typhoid, dengue, and yellow fever, Medical Department professor Hamilton Atchinson West, maintained otherwise.[21] It took a visit by John Guiteras, an official of the United States Public Health Service to settle the argument. His support of West's hypothesis was not what the locals wanted to hear. "I was down on Market Street that night after the epidemic had been declared," Howard R. Dudgeon (class of 1899) later recounted, "and even the newsboys had deserted it."[22]

The news of yellow fever in Galveston also alarmed many individuals at the Medical Department. Dudgeon remembered a few of the "more energetic" medical students "struck a bee line for the wharf and hired a little sail boat to take them across the bay to the mainland." However, rigid quarantine measures prevented the success of this and other attempts to flee the Island. Instead, one escapee later noted, students found themselves "quarantined . . . in box cars and other such delightful places."[23] While the quarantine prevented students from leaving Galveston, it kept others off. With travel to the Island suspended, J. R. Elliott (class of 1901) reported the "yellow fever scare" kept many of his classmates from matriculating. As a result, freshman enrollment that fall plummeted by almost two-thirds— from 140 to 57 students. However, many students already enrolled chose to remain at the medical school, and in the process, exhibited admirable resolve in the face of potential danger to themselves. The Medical Department senior class not only decided that classes should continue despite the epidemic, but organized a special committee to care for classmates who fell ill. Other class members provided volunteer assistance to the Board of Health.[24]

The epidemic sharpened the skills and resilience of the faculty as well. Just days before the outbreak, twenty-eight-year-old William Spencer Carter, the newly appointed head of the physiology department, arrived from Philadelphia with his young wife. Upon news of "yellow jack" on the Island, the acting dean of the medical school, Allen J. Smith, approached the freshly hired professor. "Carter," he contended, "I can't urge you to stay under the circumstances, but if you do stay, and are alive at the end of it, you will be very glad that you did so." While William Keiller remembered a newly hired chemistry professor "left Galveston by the first available train," Carter chose to stay in spite of the danger, and, as far as Keiller knew, never regretted the decision.[25] Upon succeeding Allen J. Smith as dean of the medical school in 1903, Carter championed nationally renowned research initiatives that explored the symptomology of both yellow and malarial fevers. In collaboration with Carter, Galveston city officials passed a series of sanitation ordinances, including the covering of open cisterns that considerably diminished future threats of yellow fever in Galveston.[26]

On the heels of the yellow fever epidemic, the medical school confronted another upheaval. On February 15, 1898, the tense relationship between the United States and Spain came to an explosive head with the mysterious sinking of the American battleship *Maine* in the harbor of Havana, Cuba. Two months later, the United States entered its first war in over thirty years, and the country needed volunteers. Medical Department students and recent alumni rushed to enlist, including thirty-seven from the medical school, six pharmacy students, and four from the school of nursing. Some served as surgeons in volunteer regiments while many others, particularly undergraduates, were mustered as apothecaries and hospital stewards. Because the war was of such brief duration—less than four months—very few of these enlistees saw active duty. Nevertheless, the active participation of Medical Department volunteers set the tone for greater engagement in World War I, World War II, and the Korean War.[27]

The Medical Department had much to celebrate at the dawn of the twentieth century. The school was approaching its tenth anniversary, and great hope and optimism abounded as administrators and faculty reflected upon how far the school had come in almost ten years. With the help of a determined faculty, the school had withstood financial distress, a threatening epidemic, and other crises. Throughout those difficult years Professor James Thompson recalled, "we struggled on . . . proud in the belief that we were educating doctors just as clever and capable as those coming from the best schools of the country." Up until the fall 1900 term, Thompson stated, "we had been teaching, and I say it with pride, we had been teaching well."[28] As a result of the untiring efforts of the medical school faculty, student graduates during those early years possessed the talent, stamina, and education to become genuine medical professionals. On April 22, 1892, the first three graduates of the University of Texas Medical Department, Thomas Flavin, Houston Thomas Guinn, and Jesse P. Hendrick, received their degrees during a ceremony in Galveston's Harmony Hall.[29] By 1900 the faculty had conferred medical degrees on 259 graduates. University of Texas President William Prather declared the Medical Department, having earned a reputation for high academic standards, "the best of the South."[31]

Perseverance had paid off, but as the Medical Department faculty prepared for the tenth academic session, a dangerous storm was developing in the Atlantic bearing consequences no one would foresee. In the early morning hours of Friday, September 7, 1900, the office of the Weather Bureau in Washington, D.C., issued a storm warning for the Gulf Coast from Pensacola, Florida, to Galveston, Texas. Island citizens could see the storm gradually coming in from the east. The Gulf winds increased and the surf swelled higher and higher. But very few individuals were prepared for what awaited them. In the late afternoon of September 8, a storm of catastrophic proportions slammed into the Island. Waves pulverized buildings, and rows of houses and businesses disappeared as the storm surge rose almost fifteen feet. Wind gusts measuring over 120 miles per hour ripped trees from the ground and hurled tons of debris across the Island. "All about was one continuous roar," Allen J. Smith later recounted, "the heavy sound of the rush of the wind, like one never-ending, deafening thunder, drowning the cries of the distressed, the smashing of homes and the grinding of timbers, merging them all into one indistinguishable whole."[32]

The rapid approach and brutality of the storm caught many Galveston citizens by surprise. Numerous individuals found themselves stranded from their homes and families. Some sought protection from the storm inside Old Red's massive brick walls, while John Sealy Hospital served as a haven for others. "I saw big waves go racing down the streets, and slate shingles whisked about as though they had been snowflakes, and they were nearly as thick," recalled Howard Dudgeon, an intern at the John Sealy Hospital, "windows were blown in and doors and transoms were twisted off their hinges, and at the height of the gusts the hospital building would shake like a leaf." The frightful episode frayed the nerves of even the bravest souls within the hospital, and it seemed, Dudgeon wrote, "like the very anchors of night had failed."[33] Unable to reach his home on Thirty-Fifth Street, Nicholas Clayton rode out the storm inside his Strand Street offices. Holed up in the dark, listening to the relentless screaming winds, Clayton agonized over the fate of his beloved family and his life's work.[34]

The storm began to ebb just before midnight on Saturday. As Sunday morning dawned, Clayton discovered a scene of appalling desolation. The

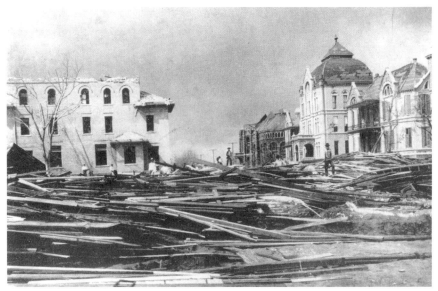

1900 storm debris. Old Red and John Sealy Hospital can be seen in the background to the right. *Courtesy Blocker History of Medicine Collections, Moody Medical Library.*

storm demolished two-thirds of Galveston's buildings and took between 6,000 and 8,000 lives. The Island was littered with bodies, many of them entrapped in a colossal pile of debris amassed by the storm that measured two stories tall and three miles in length. "No pen, nor tongue, nor painter's brush could convey anything like an adequate conception of it," wrote Columbus physician R. H. Harrison to the editor of the *Texas Medical Journal*, "the mangled remains of sea-beaten victims, the floating bodies of women with half-born babes protruding from their bodies, the shrieks and cries of the thousands of victims imprisoned beneath the great mass of wreckage . . . all made a scene of indescribable horror."[35] It was impossible, Surgeon C. T. Peckham of the United States Medical Health Service claimed, "to look upon the devastation and not weep for the lost."[36] Yet, along with the sorrow came immense relief. Every member of the Clayton family had survived. So had much of Clayton's architectural legacy, including the John Sealy Hospital and his treasured Old Red.

As the storm subsided, an anxious Dean Allen J. Smith struck out for the medical school campus. Impatient to know the fate of Old Red and the hospital, Smith waded for blocks in knee-deep water, climbing over house-high drifts of death before reaching the medical school. To his profound relief, Smith discovered Old Red still stood, badly beaten, but firmly intact. Many of Old Red's unique architectural elements were missing. Smith observed, "The ornaments of the side roofs, the cornices and gutters, the slates from nearly the whole broad covering of the building, the minaret-life caps of the ornamental pillars of the structure—all were gone or wrecked." The great dome had also collapsed, leaving a huge gap in the middle part of the roof and front wall. The storm tore the roof off the school morgue or "dead-house" and swept the building "clean of its contents." Some discoveries echoed the macabre. Smith located many of the morgue's "uncanny inhabitants, intended for the dissecting room" strewn among the rubbish, "unfit for use when opportunity came for their recovery and storage." The storm hammered or destroyed other campus buildings as well. University Hall incurred severe damage while the nurses' home was totally swept away. "Nothing was left," wrote Smith, "but a mass of drift . . . not a vestige marked the site." Happily, however, there were no casualties at the dormitory as all the student nurses found refuge within John Sealy Hospital during the early hours of the storm.[37]

Galveston had suffered the worst natural disaster in the history of the United States, but with substantial aid, the wounded city quickly began to recover. Physicians and nurses throughout the United States, including the nursing pioneer Clara Barton, traveled to the Island and volunteered their services. Newspaper mogul William Randolph Hearst railroaded in supplies. To effectively supervise civic affairs throughout the recovery and beyond, residents adopted a new commission form of city government that evolved into the city manager plan. Just five days after the storm, basic water service had been restored to the Island, and the Western Union wires were tapping telegraph messages. Within three weeks, the port of Galveston was shipping cotton out of its wharves.[38]

Over the next decade, post-storm Galveston percolated with renewal, technological innovation, and community grit. With the help of talented engineers, the city developed an ambitious plan to rebuild itself, stronger and more secure from the ravages of Mother Nature. Sturdy iron and steel bridges connected the Island to the mainland. The seawall, a six-mile-long and seventeen-feet-high concrete edifice, was designed and constructed to hold back the sea. To ensure the seawall's effectiveness, engineers executed the most amazing feat of all: a mammoth, decade-long task of raising the grade level throughout the city. For five hundred blocks, every house, building, church and school, streetcar track, fireplug, and water pipe was elevated with jackscrews, some as high as thirteen feet. The gaping spaces created underneath each structure were filled with over six million cubic yards of sand dredged from the ocean floor. Self-propelled hopper dredges transported the tons of sand along a distribution canal to stations where the loads would be pumped through pipes running down the city streets and avenues. Throughout the grade-raising process, residents navigated

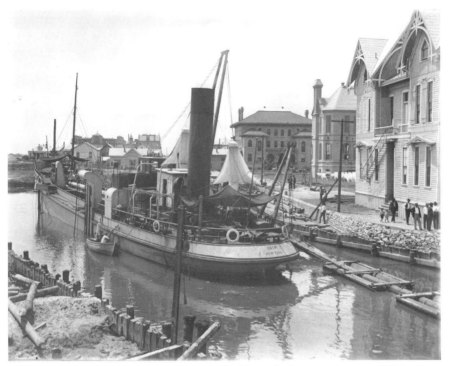

Dredge boat in a canal bordering the east end of the Medical Department campus (1904–05). Buildings pictured include left to right: St. Mary's Infirmary, far distant, University Hall, right center, and the Nurses Home, front right. *Courtesy Peabody-Essex Museum, Salem, Massachusetts.*

from place to place along elevated planks and boardwalks, some eight to ten feet high. In total, over two thousand structures of various kinds were raised throughout Galveston, including many on the eastern end of the Island where the medical school existed. Galveston had become "a city on stilts."[39]

While Old Red was spared physical elevation outright, it did not escape the logistical nightmare associated with the grade-raising project. The canal that bore dredging barges to and from the bay, wound along the eastern border of the medical school campus. Medical school faculty and students endured life among ceaseless noise, mud, and standing water. After a heavy winter rain in 1905 submerged the planked pathway to Old Red, an exasperated Dean William S. Carter exclaimed to UT President William Prather, "This grade-raising is far worse than the storm and if it were put to a vote of the people now I believe they would prefer to take the chances of another storm."[40] Carter, like many others, was undoubtedly relieved when the grade-raising project on the eastern end came to a close in 1909. By that time, Galveston's phenomenal recovery was being heralded throughout the state. "Other cities have made progress and improvements," proclaimed an anonymous advertiser in the May 1909 issue of the *Texas State Journal of Medicine*, "but it is doubtful if any other city has ever accomplished so much in such a short time."[41]

The Medical Department also experienced a historic turning point during the period immediately following the storm. Throughout its first decade, the medical school had proven itself invaluable to the people of Texas. More than four hundred physicians, pharmacists, and nurses had earned diplomas, taking their professional expertise to every region of the state. Despite this fact, the legislature and regents traditionally regarded the medical school with pecuniary ambivalence. Those attitudes began to change in the wake of the storm. The seriously battered medical school required extensive repairs. Having enjoyed the benefits of a state medical school over the past ten years, Texans strongly encouraged a quick recovery for the school. As the cheering cry, "The University of Texas stops for no storm," quickly flew across the telegraph wires, members of the Board of Regents Medical Committee, UT officials, and legislators met to fund the repairs. The delighted faculty clearly understood the significance of the action. "It was," Professor James Thompson remembered, "the first time that the regents had dipped deliberately into the available university fund to supply the needs of the Medical Department; and this very act made us feel that our school really belonged to the parent university and was not merely a stepchild."[42] The total cost was $60,000. John Sealy the younger personally financed repairs of the hospital, while the Regents Medical Committee allocated $5,000 to repair and renovate Old Red.[43]

The benevolence of the regents and Sealy provided a significant boon for the medical school. Old Red acquired a new roof complete with a large skylight that shed a broad field of natural light into the anatomy dissection lab on the third floor. Also at this time, the familiar red clay roof tile was put on to replace the colorful blue and green slate. The pharmaceutical and chemical laboratories in the basement of Old Red were completely restored and equipped, including the acquisition of new microscopes and the replacement of badly damaged instruments. Best of all, the school finally had a fully furnished and organized medical library. Located on first floor of Old Red, the new facility came complete with a librarian, Florence Magnenat, and "a suitable appropriation" to annually finance it. Thompson later declared that, by the end of the restoration, the medical school was in better shape than it had ever been.[44]

On the fifteenth of November—only two months after the storm—Old Red reopened for the fall 1900 session. With a post-storm enrollment of 119 students, the medical school faculty swelled with pride and anticipation for the future. "Like a phoenix from its fire," Professor Allen J. Smith proclaimed at the annual opening of the Medical Department in 1901, "the institution has arisen from the wreckage . . . more fully equipped in a material sense and full of the strength of the past decade's growth, calm in the reliance which triumph over difficulties and danger ever brings, a fixed part of the great educational scheme of Texas—to stay while Texas stands."[45]

Post-storm development at the school reflected the sentiments expressed by Smith. In order to grow effectively, the Medical Department broadened its services to a greater number of individuals in need. Between 1901 and 1915, several new hospitals were added to the campus that provided quality medical care for African Americans, women and children, and sufferers of infectious diseases. Patients in these facilities provided students with additional opportunities for clinical study. Built in 1901, the Negro Hospital, the first hospital for African Americans in Texas, was heralded by the *Galveston Daily News* as "one of the best buildings of its kind in the South." The newspaper praised the "well-ventilated and lighted" facility, which contained private rooms, two charity wards, and "a fine system of sanitary plumbing."[46] In January 1913, the first state hospital for physically disabled children in Texas opened its doors on the medical school campus. The Walter Colquitt Memorial Hospital, later renamed the State Hospital for Crippled and Deformed Children, was primarily established to meet the needs of children crippled by bone tuberculosis of the hip, spine, and joints.[47] To answer the necessity for better female health care facilities, the school acquired a Woman's Hospital and also built a new dormitory for nurses.

In relation to campus expansion, two enterprising deans, Allen J. Smith and William S. Carter, pushed to raise academic standards at the Medical Department. In 1910 the matriculation requirement rose to one full year of college study and two years by 1917. Carter also considered post-graduate internships an important aspect of a well-rounded medical education. In an address to the Medical Department in 1914, Carter extolled the School of Medicine as a leading institution among medical schools. As proof, he noted that every medical school graduate who wanted an internship had been able to acquire one at a hospital in the United States.[48]

The crowning achievement of Carter's lengthy term as the medical school dean involved an illustrious visitor to the Island. In an effort to align American medical standards more closely with those of Europe, the Carnegie Foundation for the Advancement of Teaching and the American Medical Association commissioned Abraham Flexner to make a thorough evaluation of medical schools throughout the United States and Canada.

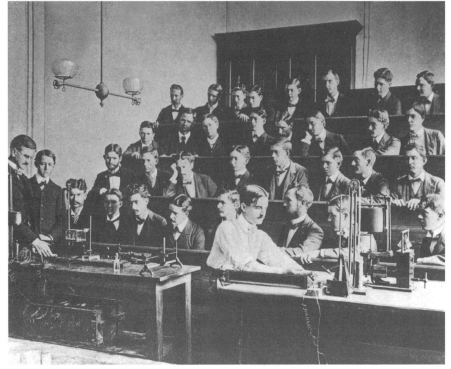

Physiology lab, Old Red. William Spencer Carter is pictured far left. *Courtesy Blocker History of Medicine Collections, Moody Medical Library.*

Flexner embarked on his monumental North American tour in January 1909. The following November, he was ascending the steps of Old Red.

Medical schools came and went in Texas during the early years of the twentieth century. Six existed in the state at the time of Flexner's visit. They included the University of Texas Medical Department (1891), the Dallas Medical College (1900), Gate City Medical College (1902), Bell Medical College (1901), Southwestern University Medical College (1903), and Baylor University College of Medicine (1903). Flexner claimed most of these a substandard lot. While each was established on charitable and humanitarian grounds, the schools were, in Flexner's words "without resources, without ideals, without facilities, though at Baylor the conjunction of hospital and laboratory might be made effective if large sums . . . were at hand."[49] Flexner found an exception in Galveston. In his classic report, *Medical Education in the United States and Canada* (1910), Flexner proclaimed the University of Texas Medical Department to be the only school in Texas "fit to continue in the work of training physicians."[50] The school housed within Old Red received high praise for its superior teaching laboratories and anatomy facilities including "a large pathological museum, labeled, and indexed," a "good" library and a university teaching hospital organized "along sound lines."[51]

Flexner was less impressed with the level of research conducted at the medical school. In his view, teaching, whether in the classroom or at the bedside, should not be the sole function of a medical school. The development of scientific knowledge was also vitally important. Several faculty members including Professors Smith and Carter, had engaged in groundbreaking research. However, Flexner either felt these projects were not enough to carry the school or ignored them. Flexner stated in his report, that there was "[n]o effort" made at the Medical Department in terms of research.[52]

American medical education felt the force of Flexner's stern evaluation. The worst or substandard schools soon disappeared, while the better ones improved. Of the six medical schools visited by Flexner on the Texas leg of his tour, only the University of Texas Medical Department and the Baylor College of Medicine survived. The Medical Department administrators glowed in the favorable rating given to the school, despite the low marks in research. Shortly after Flexner published his report, the Medical Department received an A-plus ranking from the American Medical Association's Council on Medical Education for the years 1910 and 1913. "The University of Texas had been in the first class," Dean Carter elatedly proclaimed. "May it always maintain this standing and may it continue to progress in the future as it has in the past."[53] With the addition of hospitals and ancillary facilities, the school evolved into a sophisticated health complex over the next few years. Along with the growth came a new name. In 1919 school officials replaced "Medical Department" with "Medical Branch." Since then, Old Red has presided over the University of Texas Medical Branch, or simply UTMB.[54]

Despite hard-won academic success, campus development, and a new name, the future of UTMB—and therefore Old Red—was far from secure. Since its founding, there had always been talk of moving the medical school out of Galveston. Throughout his nineteen years as dean, William Carter was continually besieged by powerful voices strongly opposed to keeping the medical school on the Island. Early UT presidents George T. Winston and William Prather supported the current location, but their successors preferred a single campus in Austin. These critics had a powerful ally in Abraham Flexner. Although UTMB received an admirable rating, Flexner noted in his report that the original decision to separate the medical school from the main university in Austin was a "regrettable mischance." If placed in Austin, Flexner believed UTMB would "gain in every way: the town is as large, and various state institutions there would strengthen its clinical opportunities; it would be easier to attract . . . outsiders in teaching positions; the stimulus of the university would assist the growth of a productive spirit." In Flexner's view, the isolation of UTMB from the parent university increased the chance of stagnation. "Perhaps," he proposed, "it is not yet too late for the people of the state to concentrate their state institutions of higher learning in one single plant."[55] However, for Carter and others at UTMB, the principal issue was money. The school's loyal and generous benefactor—the Sealy family—lived in Galveston. There was no such substitute in Austin. By 1920, Carter was waging a full-fledged battle to keep the doors of Old Red open.[56]

Mother Nature did not help Carter's case. Galveston, after all, was located on a sandbar in the Gulf of Mexico. After witnessing the incredible devastation wrought by the storm of 1900, was it wise, asked UT officials, for the medical school to remain in a location so vulnerable to destructive hurricanes? In mid-August 1915, another massive hurricane furiously descended upon Galveston, lashing the city with heavy wind and rain, and pushing the tide even higher than the 1900 storm. However, modern technology spared Galveston a repeat performance of 1900. The newly constructed seawall held throughout the storm of 1915; as a result, the storm claimed only eight lives—a great contrast to the thousands of lives lost just a few years before.

Nevertheless, hurricane winds and flying debris severely battered many architectural gems on the Island, including Old Red. In a telegram to UT President William J. Battle, the Medical Department provost, Thomas H. Nolan, provided a litany of damages to the building: "Sky lights and most of the tiling blown off college building – one hundred panes glass broken – some damage to laboratories on upper floors – laboratories in basement badly damaged by mud and water."[57] The damage to Old Red was extensive, causing some individuals to doubt the future of the institution. Upon arrival to the campus in early October 1915, C. B. Carter, a self-described "green and timid freshman," claimed that he and fellow classmate Bedford Shelmire were "greatly shocked" to find water still standing inside Old Red along with "cadavers and other debris floating in the basement." The scene resulted in long-distance telephone calls home pleading a transfer to the medical school at Tulane University—but to no avail. "Our parents were not very sympathetic," Carter recalled, "and told us to stick it out."[58] On a post-storm visit to the medical school, alumnus T. T. Jackson was struck by Old Red's "dejected" appearance. The building, he wrote, "does not look like it was a medical building of the University of the greatest State in America." To Jackson, Old Red appeared "a bit cowed and had her head hung."[59] Although the school rebounded by late spring of 1916, and Old Red was fully restored, the fiasco created by the 1915 storm strengthened the argument to move the school off the Island. While the seawall and raising the grade improved the city's safety, Galveston would always be privy to destructive hurricanes.

Another important development hindered the argument to keep UTMB in Galveston. The "Queen City of the Gulf" was losing her prominence. The oil boom, launched at Spindletop, was transforming the Gulf Coast and Texas Plains. Houston, Dallas, and many other Texas cities and towns were growing rapidly. On top of that, the United States Corps of Engineers had succeeded in dredging a deepwater thoroughfare up Buffalo Bayou to Houston. With the completion of the Houston Ship Channel in 1914, Galveston's days as the leading commercial port in Texas were numbered.[60] As more Galveston citizens departed for opportunities on the mainland, officials feared UTMB hospitals would suffer a shortage of clinical material for teaching.[61]

The drumbeat of war drew attention away from Galveston's flagging fortunes temporarily. On April 6, 1917, two years after the sinking of the British passenger liner *Lusitania*, Congress declared war on Germany and created the American Expeditionary Forces (AEF) to join the battle weary Allies on the European front. More than two million "doughboys" journeyed "over there" to fight the enemy. Almost 200,000 enlistees—including 450 female nurses—were Texans, many of whom believed their state had a special interest in the war. German foreign secretary Arthur Zimmermann's infamous offer to return lands ceded after the Treaty of Guadalupe Hidalgo in 1848 to Mexico created uneasiness within the Lone Star State. "We may find an enemy closer to us than any European power," the *Houston Post* surmised. "War upon the fields of Texas is not beyond the powers of the imagination."[62] While the threat of a German invasion—perhaps along the Texas Gulf Coast—encouraged Texans to enlist, UTMB students and alumni answered the call for volunteers on different grounds. The United States military needed doctors and lots of them. Thousands of medical volunteers were required to examine recruits, promote good hygiene among the camps, and care for the wounded.[63] "The work of the medical men in hygiene, sanitation, and in preventive medicine will help tremendously to win the present war," anatomy professor Harry O. Knight beseeched students and faculty in the fall of 1917, "There is no other profession that has more power . . . As medical men we must not hesitate to answer the call of our country."[64] By the autumn of 1918, more than 300 UTMB students and alumni entered military service, including 31 from the entering class of 1922. One of the first alumni to enlist was Dr. Ernst William Bertner (class of 1911), who joined the medical staff of John J. Pershing, supreme commander of the American Expeditionary Forces.[65]

Most medical students contributed to the war effort without ever leaving the UTMB campus. Military training came to them instead. To help protect the home front, the United States War Department organized and installed the Students Army Training Corps (SATC) or, as commonly dubbed by students, "Safe At The College." Almost every able-bodied adult male student joined up. An Army headquarters was established across the street from Old Red, with a canteen in the women's dorm, University Hall. Each morning and afternoon throughout the fall of 1918, corps members donned the reserve officer uniform, assembled on the front lawn of Old Red, and drilled under the command of United States military officers. However, such pomp and parade in the humid Galveston climate soon wore thin. Corps members, chafing over having to attend class or patients in the hospital wards directly after such hot and sweaty work, petitioned for a change in drilling hours.

Physical discomfort aside, students found wartime Galveston a thrilling place to be. "There was much going on," Howard O. Smith (class of 1922) later reflected, "foreign ships from every country were tied up at the docks and colorful uniforms of the various countries of the world could be seen on the street day or night." Interestingly, Smith noted, the international dialogue remained congenial in most cases, even on liquor-enhanced Saturday nights "when arguments about the respective merits of the various countries involved in the war arose."[66] For those who enjoyed it, the excitement of wartime in Galveston was short-lived. Germany surrendered to the Allies on November 11, 1918, less than three months after the SATC began operations on campus. Shortly afterward, the student reserve corps marched out once more to the front lawn of Old Red, folded the flags, and sounded the final retreat.

As wartime fever dissipated, UTMB faculty and administrators pitched a renewed battle to keep their school in Galveston. It hit a climax in 1920 when Abraham Flexner arrived once more on the steps of Old Red. The previous year, oil magnate and philanthropist John D. Rockefeller had donated $20 million to the General Education Board (GEB) for distribution to medical schools throughout the country. Hoping to acquire money for UTMB, Carter invited Flexner, the board's secretary, to pay a return visit to the Island. Flexner obliged and toured both UTMB and Baylor College of Medicine in Dallas. The enthusiastic citizens of Dallas had raised half a million dollars for new facilities at their medical school, while Baylor University pledged $1 million. Flexner was impressed with the improvements made to Baylor and recommended a $300,000 allocation by the GEB to the school. He was not impressed by UTMB. Galveston city officials, balking at the cost of care for indigent patients at John Sealy Hospital lost interest in renewing the hospital and tightened its purse

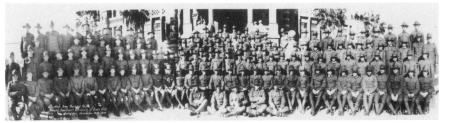

Student Army Training corps at the Medical Department, 1918. The Corps was active from October to December 1918. During that brief period of time, student members of the corps wore khaki uniforms and drilled with wooden guns. *Courtesy Blocker History of Medicine Collections, Moody Medical Library.*

strings. For the fiscal year 1921, the city commissioners slashed funding to John Sealy Hospital by two-thirds from $30,000 to $10,000. Flexner doubted the medical school could truly develop without controlling its own hospital and thus, to Carter's disappointment, UTMB was denied any Rockefeller funds.[67]

In comparing the institution to thriving Baylor, critics predicted UTMB had little chance of survival. "Galveston," regent W. H. Dougherty declared, "is dead."[68] In June 1920, the George R. Hermann estate in Houston, the benefactor of many scientific and philanthropic endeavors, became interested in funding the relocation of the school to a site near Houston's Rice Institute. The motion was known as the Tillotson Resolution in the Texas House. Investigating the matter, Governor William Hobby appointed a committee to look into "the advisability of removing the Medical Branch to some other city in the State," most likely the Bayou City.[69]

The gesture was strongly supported by UT President Robert E. Vinson, an ardent advocate of relocation. In the midst of hearings organized by the governor's committee in November 1920, Vinson testified to the physical inadequacy of the UTMB campus, the negotiating headaches with city commissioners, the declining number of hospital inpatients for clinical teaching, and the subsequent lack of research initiatives. "I have no desire," Vinson heatedly asserted during testimony, "to be president of a third class jack-leg medical college."[70] The deck appeared stacked against keeping the school in Galveston. However, the release of the governor's committee report in December told a different story. According to the state attorney general, since the selection of Galveston as the location for the medical school had been decided by popular vote, neither the legislature nor the University of Texas Board of Regents had the power to relocate UTMB without "the discretion of the people."[71] The oldest medical school in the state would stay put. The Tillotson Resolution had been defeated. In its place, the governor's committee recommended that John Sealy Hospital become a fully funded state hospital and improvements be made to the physical campus. The relocation crisis had finally passed—at least for the time being. While underlying political tensions remained, two decades would elapse before another battle to transfer the medical school out of Galveston would arise.

The 1920s and 1930s were a dynamic period for Galveston and UTMB, as both the city and medical school embraced new directions and opportunities. As Houston with its thriving Ship Channel continued to outpace Galveston economically, many business interests on the Island changed course, fervently pursuing the tourist trade. For decades, Galveston had attracted visitors with its beaches, hotels, and entertainment venues. However, by the early 1920s, the increasing popularity of automobiles and the construction of all-weather roads made it easier for individuals to visit the Island. And they did. As a tourist mecca, Galveston was hard to beat. Celebrations, festivals, and recreational events were held year-round to maintain a steady flow of tourist revenue. Visitors flocked to Mardi Gras festivities and the Oleander Fete, a spring rite commemorating the Island's celebrated flower. The most popular event was Splash Day, which marked the opening of the summer season. The celebration featured parades, dances, and beauty contests, most notably the Bathing Girl Review, which at its height attracted crowds of 250,000 people.[72]

For its own purposes, the UTMB community eagerly boosted Galveston's image as the ultimate place for fun and relaxation. Such a reputation not only attracted visitors to the Island, but also the medical school. In 1928 the school used the slogan, "Galveston: Where the World Comes to Play" to head a multi-photo advertisement in the *Texas State Journal of Medicine* heralding the Island as the location for the upcoming annual meeting of the Texas State Medical Association.[73]

Although the tourism industry thrived in Galveston, it did not keep the city afloat by itself. An active port, the Fort Crockett military base, and deep-pocketed insurance companies secured the economic well-being of the Island, especially during the Great Depression. Thanks to the creation of the Sealy and Smith Foundation, another primary asset to Galveston involved the presence of a financially viable UTMB. In 1922, distressed by the recent relocation threat and the difficulty in acquiring adequate funding from the city government for the John Sealy Hospital, John Sealy the younger paid a visit to the Rockefeller Foundation offices in New York City. His aim was to glean as much information as possible regarding the organization and implementation of endowing foundations. After careful study, Sealy and his sister, Jennie Sealy Smith, chartered the Sealy

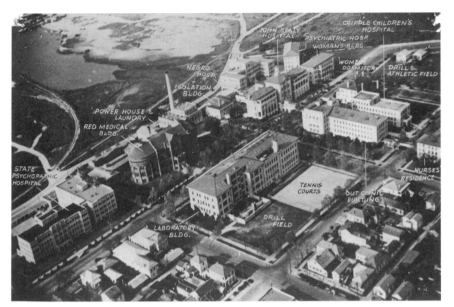

Aerial view of UTMB campus buildings, 1939. *Courtesy Rosenberg Library.*

and Smith Foundation to meet the financial needs of the hospital, including construction, renovations, expansion, and the purchase of equipment and furniture. Most importantly, interest from the endowment could only be used to directly support patient care, especially that of indigents. The move assured UTMB's future. From 1926 to 1940, the foundation directors bestowed more than $2 million on the hospital.[74]

The generosity of private donors was also highly important to UTMB throughout the 1920s and 1930s. Energetic women's groups hosted fundraisers. The Hospital Aid Society sold pencils at ten cents apiece, Red Cross Christmas Seals, and valentines to raise money for furniture, linens, toys, and other needs. By 1938 the organization had given more than $50,000 to UTMB. Private money also supported academic programs and scholarships. In addition to his ongoing support of University Hall, George Breckinridge donated money for teaching fellowships. In 1921 and 1922, Professor Marvin Graves helped finance three junior faculty positions in the Department of Medicine. Houston lawyer and businessman Will C. Hogg bequeathed $25,000 of his estate for student loans; and, in the depths of the Depression, Mrs. H. L. Ziegler of Galveston gave $2,000 to be distributed among the "most needy" members of the graduating classes of 1934 and 1935.[75]

The fattening of UTMB's coffers—whether from foundation grants, private sources, or state funds—bolstered the dreams and aspirations of faculty and administrators. Although Old Red remained at the heart of the campus, the medical school became the picture of expansion and development. Seven new buildings were added between 1923 and 1942. The Laboratory Building, later renamed the Keiller Building, provided an updated haven for the teaching of the ancillary sciences. While the freshman anatomy dissecting lab remained on the third floor of Old Red, the rest of the anatomy department, the medical school library, and administrative offices had moved out of the old landmark and into this new facility. The resultant vacancies inside Old Red were quickly filled with laboratories for microbiology, biochemistry, and physiology. The campus also acquired an Outpatient Clinic Building (1930), the forty-eight-bed Galveston State Psychopathic Hospital (1931), and a second Rebecca Sealy Nurses Home (1932), built large enough to provide spacious living quarters and house the John Sealy Training School for Nurses.[76]

New Deal funding also made a positive impact, as two replacement hospitals opened their doors in 1937. The Children's Hospital, funded by the Public Works Administration (PWA) and the Texas Legislature, sported many contemporary features including a therapeutic pool, massage rooms, and a diet kitchen. Patients and staff at the new Negro Hospital, also funded by PWA dollars, moved into a comfortable, ninety-two-bed facility that included a small ward for disabled African American children, wards for obstetrics, gynecology, and surgery. Totaling over $128,000, the PWA grant to the hospital was considered at the time to be the largest federal endowment ever received by an institution in Texas.[77]

New Deal enthusiasm at UTMB reached its peak in May of 1937 when President Franklin Delano Roosevelt made a personal visit to the school. Medical Branch officials proudly escorted Roosevelt to view the Children's and Negro Hospitals in an automobile tour of the campus. Throngs of students, faculty, caregivers, and patients lined up along the thoroughfare to greet the president's cavalcade as it slowly proceeded down the Strand, past dormitories, laboratory buildings, hospitals, and finally at the end of the street, Old Red. What was Roosevelt's reaction upon seeing the august red brick building? His thoughts, unfortunately, went unrecorded. However, being the intellectually curious man that he was, Roosevelt undoubtedly paused to acknowledge the architectural beauty and historic significance of Old Red as the touring car slowly proceeded past.[78]

Little did the crowds at UTMB realize as they celebrated the presidential visit that the medical school was about to enter the most tumultuous period of its history. In the 1940s and the 1950s, the Medical Branch confronted the demands of World War II and the Korean War, braved the

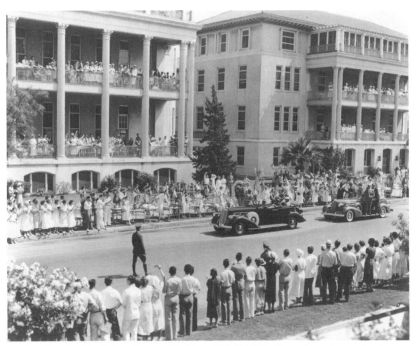

President Franklin Delano Roosevelt's visit to UTMB, 1937. Photo shows the cars bearing Roosevelt and his entourage as they pass the Woman's Hospital (right) and the old John Sealy Hospital. *Courtesy Blocker History of Medicine Collections, Moody Medical Library.*

ravages of two hurricanes, and mustered its resources to aid the survivors of the Texas City Disaster. It was also a period of new beginnings as the school overcame extraordinary political challenges to become one of the leading medical institutions in the nation.

The worst trouble began in 1938 when John Spies became dean and chief executive officer of the medical school. The UTMB deanship had changed hands several times throughout the 1920s and 1930s. After William Spencer Carter stepped down in 1922, William Keiller (1922–26), Henry Hartman (1926–28), and George Bethel (1928–35) all served a term as dean. When Bethel died in office, Carter was persuaded to return as dean for three more years (1935–38). By the autumn of 1938, John Spies had been hired as Carter's replacement. A native-born Texan who had grown up in Fannin County, Spies possessed an impressive and promising résumé: a bachelor's degree from the University of Texas, a medical diploma from the Harvard School of Medicine, plus two additional years of study in Belgium, surgical experience in New York hospitals, and academic positions at the Yale School of Medicine and Peking Union Medical College in China.[79]

In spite of his glowing credentials, Spies quickly made enemies at UTMB. One particular adversary was the man responsible for hiring Spies in the first place: Edward Randall, president of the UT Board of Regents and a professor at the medical school. Described as "irascible, arrogant and domineering," the seventy-eight-year-old Randall had a heavy hand in the city's hospital-medical school complex.[80] After going around the faculty search committees to ensure Spies's appointment, Randall presumed the new dean would be "his man" regarding any changes or developments involving the medical school. But Spies—who personally favored relocating UTMB to Houston—thought otherwise. The new dean viewed his appointment as a mandate from University of Texas President Homer P. Rainey and the regents to wrest political power out of the hands of Galveston professors and bind the medical school more tightly under university management. In Spies's mind, any tactics that helped accomplish this mission were on the table.[81]

In January 1939, John Spies arrived to begin his new position at the Medical Branch. Perhaps no one was prepared for what happened next. Spies immediately ordered the wires of the main UTMB switchboard be tapped and installed a secret tape recorder in his office. He began holding secret meetings, approved a radical reorganization of academic departments, and combined them without consulting the department chairs. Some believed Spies's actions were necessary to bring about change in a deeply rooted academic network. Spies supported university control of John Sealy Hospital, better education for nursing students, and believed academic research—an area Abraham Flexner found wanting at UTMB in his 1910 report—should be a primary goal of the medical school. However, ardent critics of Spies smelled a dictatorship. Faculty and students became divided amongst each other. It has even been suggested that Spies recruited students as spies to keep him informed about various individuals on campus, especially faculty.[82] Before the year was out, UTMB was entangled in a vicious internal war that lasted almost three years. The furious opposition slung the mud, claiming Spies was "immoral, dictatorial, professionally incompetent, verbally abusive, responsible for the suicides of two faculty members, a sex pervert, a thief, an Anti-Semitic Fascist, a communist, a Nazi sympathizer, a homosexual," and conducted "lecherous behavior" with the wives of former colleagues.[83]

By early 1942, the political infighting had become so appalling that the Texas Legislature sent a delegation, accompanied by Texas Rangers, to Galveston for the purpose of rooting out possible un-American activities or subversives at the medical school. Heart specialist Denton A. Cooley, who was a student at UTMB at the time, later described the hearings as "a kangaroo court type of investigation . . . that pitted our highly respected faculty members against one another . . . [where] many petty differences were aired before the student body."[84] Less than a week after the hearings, the legislative committee released their conclusions. The committee found no evidence of un-American activities at UTMB except a "failure to devote full efforts to training and production of doctors." While the committee recommended that Spies be dismissed, it laid much blame at the door of the regents for "permitting the present condition to grow and exist." The regents, the committee asserted, were responsible for the "decline and disrepute of the Medical Branch."[85] In May 1942, the Association of American Medical Colleges (AAMC) and the American Medical Association (AMA) put UTMB on probation. Expressing their fury that the controversy had been allowed to digress to such an extent, UTMB students held a lynching party and hung Dean Spies, UT President Rainey, and a UT regent in effigy from telephone wires within sight of Old Red.[86] The whole episode gave UTMB a serious black eye, leaving Cooley and others extremely discouraged regarding the future of the medical school. In fact, Cooley later admitted the incident triggered his decision to finish his medical studies at Johns Hopkins.[87]

The probation period at UTMB did not last long. Both the AAMC and the AMA lifted the probation in September 1943, a little more than a year after its initial enforcement. Chauncey D. Leake, who succeeded Spies as dean in the fall of 1942, was instrumental in steering UTMB to better days. An internationally renowned pharmacologist and philosopher, Leake came to Galveston after a fourteen-year stint at the University of California School of Medicine in San Francisco. As executive vice-president and dean, Leake was one of the first PhDs to serve as dean of an American medical school, and the only non-physician to hold that post at UTMB. Tall, tanned, with a thick mop of white hair, Leake arrived on campus brimming with energy, intelligence, and insight. "Couldn't be a greater contrast than that between San Francisco and Galveston," Leake wrote a friend. "Galveston is flat, hot and quite quaint. Whatever cultural activities exist must be from within. It is a proud place." Yet Leake clearly understood the extraordinary problems at UTMB and was up to the challenge. "So far it's been nothing but heat, hard work, and confusion here," he wrote another friend. But, Leake admitted, he was enjoying his new work "immensely." "Believe me," he declared, "it's something when 'the eyes of Texas are upon you.'" During his thirteen-year tenure at UTMB, Leake instituted reforms, recruited distinguished faculty, was a strong supporter of research, the expansion of academic programs on campus, and actively solicited funding from federal and private agencies. Moreover, Leake's characteristic warmth and openness was conducive to helping restore the school's traditional harmony and small-town values.[88]

During the first years of his tenure, the challenges facing Leake were not all local. America, by that time, was deeply engaged in another world war. Thomas O. Shindler recalled that, on December 7, 1941, a radio program featuring the New York City Philharmonic was interrupted to announce the Japanese attack on Pearl Harbor. "A number of us in the fraternity house were listening to the program," Schindler remembered. Following the announcement, "scarcely a word was said, with perhaps the quiet inner knowledge, unadmitted, that the war would sooner or later involve us personally."[89] And it did. Throughout World War II, the Medical Branch endured routine blackouts, the distraction of military blimps in search of enemy submarines in Gulf waters, and secret, nighttime visits to John Sealy Hospital by wounded sailors of sunken cargo vessels. No one was allowed on the beach after sundown, and a military installation occupied the eastern portion of the seawall.[90] A war being fought overseas seemed very close, indeed.

The floors and stairwells of Old Red groaned under the continuous stream of wartime activity and preparation. The rapid military buildup of the United States armed forces required the commitment of over 70,000 physicians and surgeons. Officials anticipated the U.S. land forces would reach seven million. Physicians were needed at a rate of one per every thousand soldiers. "Everything seemed more urgent," Schindler recalled, "and we were planning, each of us, the area of service we should most prefer."[91] To effectively answer the call to duty, UTMB established in 1941 an "accelerated" training program for the medical and nursing schools. Instead of classes being held for eight to nine months over a four-year period, they were conducted for eleven months over three years. More than one freshman class was admitted per year, resulting in more than one graduation ceremony as well. To complete their coursework, students crammed into lecture halls and laboratory spaces inside Old Red and other campus facilities. As a result of the academic speed-up, the Medical Branch annually launched more than one hundred physicians, while the school of nursing graduated more than fifty nurses per year.[92]

Another wartime measure involved the congressional passage in 1942 of a Student War Loan Program. Under this legislation, full-time medical students could receive low-interest loans if they agreed to enlist in the armed forces. Specialized army and navy training programs began with each new school session. This offering allowed students to continue their studies while simultaneously training to join the medical corps of the armed forces. The program required training in a variety of disciplines including map reading, field sanitation, and defense against air, gas, and

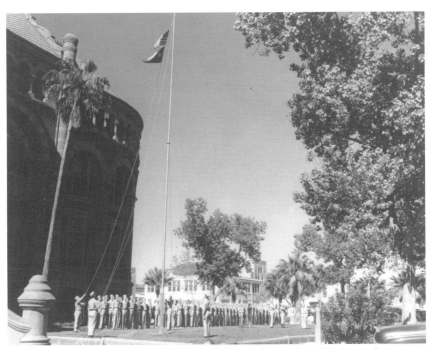

Flag-raising ceremony, Old Red, World War II. *Courtesy Blocker History of Medicine Collections, Moody Medical Library.*

mechanized attack. Students were provided with uniforms, equipment, and a $50 monthly allowance—the same allotment as that received by a U.S. army regular.[93] It was a popular venture. By the summer of 1943, almost 250 medical underclassmen—approximately 75 percent—were enrolled in either the army or navy program. In addition, twenty-nine female nursing students had enlisted in a separate specialized program.[94]

The training of physicians and nurses carried over into the creation of military medical units at UTMB. Shortly after the Japanese bombing of Pearl Harbor, the regents approved the formation of a surgical hospital unit at the Medical Branch. UTMB faculty, alumni, and other Texas physicians joined the 30th Evacuation Hospital, led by Houston physician Donald Payton. Heading overseas in late 1943, the unit, comprised of over forty professionals, received a citation for distinguished work during its two years of service in New Guinea.[95] A larger enterprise, the General Military Hospital Unit, was created at UTMB during the spring of 1942. This outfit became part of the 127th General Hospital, a 1,000-bed unit, staffed by approximately 200 medical professionals, including Medical Branch faculty and alumni. UTMB professors Truman G. Blocker

Jr., Robert Moore, and William Ainsworth joined the unit, as did alumni Carroll Adriance (class of 1940), Norman Duren (class of 1938), and Captain Grace Decker (class of 1929), an officer in the Army Nurse Corps. After seven months in southwest England, the 127th crossed the English Channel and followed the Allies in their rapid drive into France. It was the only American hospital in central and eastern Brittany during the Allies' major D-Day offensive.[96] Shortly after the Japanese surrender, Chief Surgeon of the European Theater Paul R. Hawley commended the 127th for its "inexhaustible" talent and "high standard of professional care." "It is easy," Hawley declared, "for the University of Texas to be proud of the 127th General Hospital." UTMB faculty and alumni had rendered themselves invaluable to the American cause.[97]

If the burdens involved with academic probation and wartime mobilization were not enough, two more hurricanes struck Galveston during the war years, severely damaging portions of UTMB. On the morning of July 27, 1943, a "surprise" hurricane—one of the fiercest storms ever to hit the Texas Gulf Coast—slammed into Galveston Island. Due to orders from the federal government, only a blurb appeared in the local newspapers warning of its approach. News of a potentially debilitating hurricane in the vicinity of fuel-producing refineries in Baytown and Texas City could fall into enemy hands, threatening the welfare of the United States and its allies. Therefore, few individuals—including those at the medical school—were prepared for the vicious 132-mile-per-hour winds that lashed the Island. According to one observer, the Children's Hospital shook with a cannon-like roar as the eye of the hurricane approached Galveston. Windows shattered throughout the wards and tiles "flew from the hospital like leaves." Flying timber crashed through the windows of Old Red, wrecking laboratory equipment and glassware, while water poured into the first floor. The central portion of John Sealy Hospital also became a scene of bedlam as skylights fell, plaster dropped from the ceilings, and a river of water rushed down the stairs.[98]

UTMB faculty, students, and staff briskly confronted the immediate crisis. Members of the army and navy training units evacuated hospital wards and operating rooms. Barefoot doctors delivered babies by candlelight in the Woman's Hospital, while staff waiting out the storm in other buildings banded together and sang songs to ease their nerves and pass the time. The storm continued with unabated fury until late in the afternoon. As the storm departed the Island for the mainland, Galveston citizens emerged from their shelters to assess the damage. The UTMB campus had been severely hit. University Hall, the home for women medical students for four decades, was damaged beyond repair. Classrooms and laboratory spaces within Old Red, the Keiller Building, and other facilities were immersed in water, shattered glass, broken equipment, and debris. Many buildings were missing roofs. The storm blew off many of Old Red's terra-cotta tiles and destroyed skylights on the top floor. The UTMB campus was not the only area smashed by the storm. Throughout Galveston and the mainland, the hurricane claimed twenty lives, injured hundreds more, and caused millions of dollars in property damage.[99] In August 1945, another unwelcome storm swept over the Island; but this time, UTMB was lucky. "This reports to you that the hurricane of August 27 did no damage to the Medical Branch," wrote Chauncey Leake to UT President T. S. Painter, "Student and staff morale was very high, and the experience was a helpful lesson to us all in preparation to meet disaster."[100] Thankfully, it would turn out, this storm would be the last major hurricane to hit the Island and UTMB for almost twenty years.

By the time Leake delivered his upbeat message to Painter, UTMB was celebrating far more than pull-

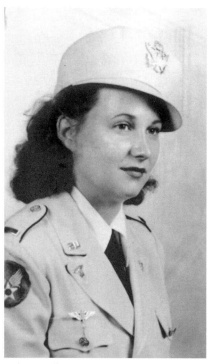

Wilma "Dolly" Vinsant. A 1940 graduate of the University of Texas School of Nursing, Vinsant was killed on an air force evacuation mission in 1943. *Courtesy Blocker History of Medicine Collections, Moody Medical Library.*

ing through another hurricane. By late August of 1945, both Germany and Japan had surrendered to the Allies. World War II was over. UTMB faculty and alumni who had joined the armed forces returned to their previous occupations. But not everyone came back. At least ten graduates of the medical and nursing schools lost their lives in World War II. One was Wilma ("Dolly") Vinsant (class of 1940), a member of the Army Nurse Corps who joined the Air Force's aeromedical evacuation program in 1943. This program successfully used flight nurses to transfer the wounded from the front lines to hospitals, thereby increasing the survival rate of armed servicemen. Headquartered in England, Vinsant completed numerous dangerous evacuation missions before her plane was shot down over Germany. When an eight-building dormitory complex was opened on the UTMB campus in 1955 and 1956, Vinsant Hall, a female dormitory, was named in her honor.[101]

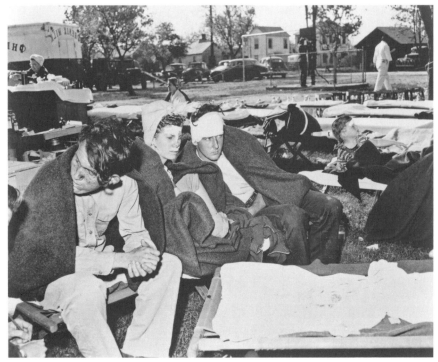

Victims of the Texas City Explosion, April 1947. *Courtesy Blocker History of Medicine Collections, Moody Medical Library.*

For the faculty and alumni who did return, service on the front and in military hospitals proved to be an invaluable experience. During the war, the American medical community was introduced to new therapeutics, including penicillin and the sulfa drugs, learned more effective treatments for trauma, and developed better skills for evacuating the wounded. As a result, UTMB physicians and caregivers emerged from the war better equipped to cope with a wide range of emergencies. Within a very short time, that expertise would be needed.[102]

Shortly after nine o'clock on the morning of April 16, 1947, UTMB encountered the deadliest manmade disaster of the twentieth century. As surgeons at John Sealy Hospital began their morning procedures, a terrific blast shook the corridors and operating rooms, causing medical instruments to jump a foot in the air. Along the Texas City docks just north of Galveston, the SS *Grandcamp*, a French freighter loaded with 2,300 tons of ammonium nitrate, exploded and devastated the expansive Monsanto chemical plant and much of the surrounding area. Sixteen hours later, a second ship carrying ammonium, the SS *High Flyer,* detonated. The subsequent reverberations knocked people to the ground in Galveston twelve miles away, shattered windows in Houston forty miles away, and rattled a seismograph in Denver, Colorado. A nurse at John Sealy Hospital remembered the blast made "a terrific noise" and "our hospital literally shook." Surgeons in the hospital operating rooms testified that instruments jumped a foot off the table.[103] The accident claimed more than six hundred lives, and an additional eight hundred required hospitalization. Three-quarters of these were sent to John Sealy.

As a cascade of ambulances roared into Galveston, UTMB doctors and nurses, many of them familiar with mass casualties of war, mobilized to meet the emergency. Ten operating teams were set up in imitation of those of military units, each composed of three to four men. For two days straight, surgeons labored

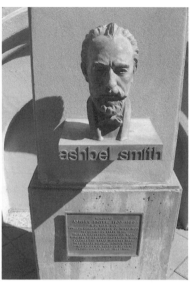

Ashbel Smith bust and plaque. A creation of Galveston sculptor Joseph Panderewski, this bust of Ashbel Smith and accompanying plaque is located at the ground floor entrance of Old Red. *Courtesy Blocker History of Medicine Collections, Moody Medical Library.*

around the clock setting fractures and repairing deep lacerations. Medical Branch students formed rescue teams and assumed other tasks dependent upon their level of training.[104] The large number of wounded inundated the hospital emergency rooms and overflowed into the building corridors. The hospital's supply of plasma—two years' worth—quickly became depleted. Dr. Dorothy Annette Cato, then an intern at John Sealy, vividly remembered that just when the hospital operating room was down to the last bottle, another stock arrived by military aircraft. Used empty plasma bottles littered the hospital. "It looked," Cato recalled, "as if a gigantic orgy had taken place."[105] Within a week, the entire reserve of newly manufactured penicillin in the United States was apportioned to Galveston.[106]

When he saw through his surgery room window a huge mushroom cloud emanating from the Texas City wharves, UTMB surgeon Truman Blocker initially feared the beginning of another global conflict. As massive numbers of casualties entered the doors of John Sealy Hospital, Blocker, then chief of maxillofacial surgery, quickly organized his staff and triaged patients with serious burns and lacerations. The experience gained that day laid the groundwork for what became a center of excellence for the treatment of burn victims: The Blocker Burn Unit, an integral part of the current Shriners Burns Institute, located on the UTMB campus.[107]

As the Texas City crisis subsided, many accident victims left John Sealy Hospital grateful for their lives. The medical school also benefited. The intuitive, professional response to the disaster by caregivers at John Sealy both affirmed UTMB's reputation as a quality institution and haven for the afflicted.

The time had come to give Old Red an official name. Almost six decades had passed since Dean J. F. Y. Paine proudly declared his dreams for the University of Texas Medical Department. During those years, Old Red welcomed and sheltered generations of aspiring students and dedicated faculty, bore witness to academic triumphs and failures, and continually withstood the wrath of Mother Nature. As the UTMB campus continued to grow and develop throughout the 1940s, there came a desire to pay homage to the place where it had all begun. On the afternoon of June 10, 1949, UTMB faculty and alumni gathered on the front lawn of Old Red to dedicate the building in honor of Ashbel Smith, medical pioneer, humanitarian, statesman, and ardent founder of the University of Texas and its medical school. The ceremony included the unveiling of a bronze bust of Smith, created by Galveston sculptor Joseph Panderewski.[108] The beautifully mounted sculpture was placed in a prominent position at the building entrance, where it remains to the current day. Since the day of dedication, the unbridled spirit of Ashbel Smith greets all who enter Old Red.

Chapter 4

STUDENT LIFE

STUDENT LIFE INSIDE OLD RED was dynamic from the beginning. Each year, the University of Texas Medical Department (later called the University of Texas Medical Branch, or UTMB) welcomed a fresh batch of pupils to three separate schools: the School of Medicine, the School of Pharmacy, and the School of Nursing. Throughout the first fifty years, Old Red served as the academic centerpiece of each program. Within its halls, students regularly attended lectures and demonstrations, conducted laboratory work, worried over grades, and at times engaged in classroom mischief to let off steam. Students at the medical school forged a vibrant community bonded by experiences unique to obtaining a medical education in Galveston.

The first classes of students at UTMB had a great deal in common. Most were young, unmarried Texans between seventeen and twenty-one years of age. The vast majority came from rural areas or small towns. Many were cash-strapped and supported themselves working on campus or took summer jobs at the Galveston docks, clerked in drugstores, sold magazines, or were employed at other local ventures.[1]

An unusual feature of these first classes involved the acceptance of female students. The nursing school admitted only women, but the schools of medicine and pharmacy were coeducational from the start. Although this arrangement was not uncommon—at least forty medical schools across the United States in the 1890s claimed a female student body of 10 percent or more—UTMB was still exceptional. Most regular medical schools during this period practiced gender segregation, while female medical and pharmacy students at UTMB took all of their classes alongside their male classmates.[2]

Living arrangements varied. Female medical and pharmacy students lived in boardinghouses until the opening of University Hall in 1898. In hopes of encouraging more young Texas women to study medicine, UT regent and philanthropist George W. Brackenridge anonymously donated $41,000 for their residence hall. Constructed of cream-colored brick and

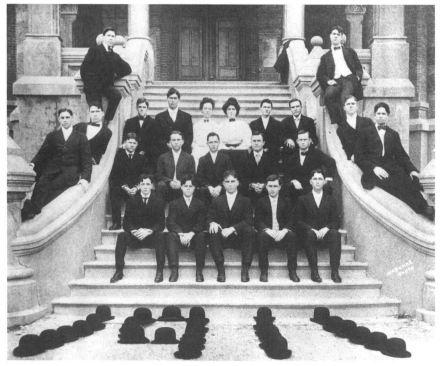

Medical Department Class of 1911. Note the hats are arranged to form "1911." *Courtesy Blocker History of Medicine Collections, Moody Medical Library.*

terra-cotta, the beautiful thirty-bedroom dormitory housed female students until it was demolished in the 1950s. Male students, on the other hand, resided wherever they could: rooming houses, spare bedrooms, or apartments scattered throughout Galveston.

Nursing students had a different setup. During the early years, the Nurses Home was a gingerbread-framed structure that formerly housed the old City Hospital and later the Texas Medical College. In the early years, the Negro Hospital occupied the first floor while the nurses lived on the second. This arrangement continued until the completion of a new Negro Hospital in 1901. When the patients moved out, the nursing school had command of the entire building. One portion was used as a residence hall and the other for classroom space. In 1915 student nurses got their own full-fledged dormitory: the ornate Rebecca Sealy Nurses' Home, beautifully constructed of stucco in the Italian Renaissance style.

Regardless of their residential habitats, all students departed for classes each day dressed in the customary uniform. For female medical and pharmacy students, proper attire consisted of a high-collared shirtwaist and dark skirt. Males wore a light wool suit complete with vest, tie, and derby hat. The original uniform for student nurses included a blue ankle-length dress, with white linen cuffs, a white bib and apron, and a white linen cap.[3]

Many of the early students shared one additional characteristic: they were woefully unprepared for the rigors of a medical education. Modest funding from the state legislature during the early years forced UTMB to rely upon student fees to cover the school's operating costs. Compelled to compete with less credible schools for students, UTMB initially upheld only the basic requirements for admission. Although faculty preference was given to applicants possessing a high school or college diploma, aspiring medical students could enroll as long as they passed examinations in elementary spelling, grammar, and physics. The admission policies were similar for the pharmacy school. Applicants to that line of study were required to write a three hundred-word essay and pass an elementary mathematics exam. "Perhaps one of our most serious handicaps was the poor preparation of our students," UTMB Professor of Anatomy William Keiller later reflected, "as we had to adapt ourselves to the state of general education in Texas at the time in selecting our medical students."[4]

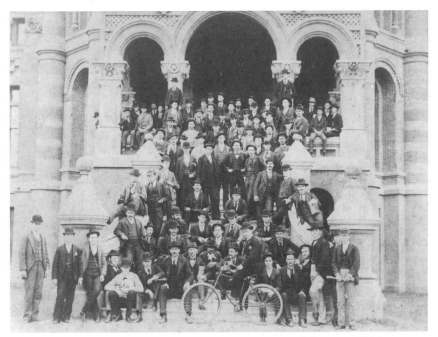

Early student group on the steps of Old Red (1894–95). *Courtesy Blocker History of Medicine Collections, Moody Medical Library.*

By 1897 the UTMB faculty required applicants without diplomas to pass an entrance examination akin to that given under similar circumstance at the University of Texas in Austin. As for the School of Nursing, Katherine Gonder Lovelady (class of 1899) recalled, "Admission in those days required only the ability to read and write and have common sense."[5] While a basic elementary education was all the academic preparation needed to enter the nursing school, other conditions also applied. Nursing students were required to possess a strong moral character, good health, and be between nineteen and thirty-five years of age. It was not until 1927 that the first nursing class composed entirely of high school graduates entered UTMB, three years before the state of Texas required a high school diploma for admission.[6]

While getting into UTMB could be relatively simple during the early years, staying there was another matter. Determined to retain high standards of scientific achievement in their graduates, the UTMB faculty set a demanding curriculum for its students. The first-year medical schedule included courses in anatomy, physiology, chemistry and physics, drugs and therapeutics, pathology—as well as a lab for each. Subsequent terms were equally challenging. Second- and third-year students attended a wholesale series of lectures and lab courses and received clinical instruction in the hospital wards. They also had an anatomical dissection lab every evening from Monday through Friday. Weekends were booked as well. There were clinics and operative gynecology on Saturday mornings and a chemistry lab on Saturday afternoons. In the fall of 1897, the faculty added another full year to the medical school program and lengthened the annual term from seven to eight months.[7]

From their very first day of medical school, aspiring practitioners became immersed in a daunting routine that left many rattled and perplexed. In his memoir, J. Gordon Bryson (class of 1910) recalled how quickly his freshman enthusiasm deflated upon assuming his seat for the first time in William Keiller's anatomy lab. "All freshmen were issued a pouch of little bones of either the hand or foot with ankle and wrist, depending upon your section," wrote Bryson. "From anatomy we went to histology for two hours. The afternoon started with two hours of chemistry lab, followed by an hour lecture each on materia medica and physiology. The first day could not have been more confusing to me had I been in China being taught the *Origin of the Species* by an Italian who spoke German."[8] One student compared the medical school experience to a baseball game. Those who survive "must hit the ball from the start," and remain on the run for the next four years.[9] Days crammed full with class and lab work were usually followed by long evenings of intense study. "It is significant that the labs are never locked," noted Willard R. Cooke (class of 1912), " for one rarely passes the college at night that he does not see lights blazing away until the small hours."[10]

Adding to the stress, many early medical students encountered derision from the local populace. Galveston society in general viewed medical students as unwelcome visitors to endure for a time. As the students trudged to and from campus often carrying skulls and bones to study, teenage street toughs harassed them yelling "Yeah, bone jugglers, bone jugglers!" in hopes of being chased. Other citizens explicitly feared the young physicians-in-training. Some African American parents warned their children to be home by dark for fear the medical students would abduct them for experiments.[11]

Many UTMB students did not last long in the program. A series of rigid examinations given by the medical school faculty weeded out the academically unfit. And the weeding was ruthless. Before 1906, when the American Medical Association raised the standards of admission into medical school to include a high school diploma, 50 to 70 percent of each entering medical school class failed or were "busted" out. Beginning with the first UTMB medical school class of twenty-three students, fourteen remained a few weeks into the fall semester of 1891, and only twelve of those students made it to graduation. The Schools of Pharmacy and Nursing were also extremely challenging. On average, half of the students admitted the first year survived each program to enroll for the second. Less than half made it to graduation at the end of the second year. Other students left on their own accord, some transferring to other medical schools. Tulane University in New Orleans was a favorite second choice for many who found UTMB too difficult.[12]

The astounding attrition rate sobered many students to the grim realities of medical school. Practically every student lived in dread of the utter humiliation and disappointment associated with failing. Giving voice to these fears was an everlasting theme in student publications, including the University of Texas system yearbook, the *Cactus*. While proud of the successful completion of their degrees, the class of 1897 straightforwardly noted in their senior *Cactus*: "eighty four strong, this class began its career in October, '94. Since that time, more than one half have fallen by the wayside." In the same yearbook, young scribes in the class of 1898 penned the following theatrical lyric to express their sentiments:

It was no plague, no pestilence, naught in which the grim visaged monster played a part, that caused this thinning of the ranks.
Twas the deadly scourging work of the demon chemistry, the fiend histology and the anatomy devil.[13]

Perhaps one of the most creative entries in the *Cactus* was submitted in 1905 when a remorseful student penned this rendition of the sixteenth-century Cardinal Thomas Wolsey's reputed last words: "Would to God I had served my books as I have the nurses; they would not have deserted me."[14] The *University Medical,* a student publication that featured news and articles from alumni, frequently supplied advice on keeping academically afloat. Editorials offered guidance regarding the best methods of taking notes, study habits, and preparing for exams. The journal also issued warnings regarding the wholesale use of stimulants from caffeine to strychnine. In 1896 two students reported that they studied botany from 9 p.m. until 6 a.m. the next morning, and they recommended "Muscat Mineral Water" over caffeine for the nerves.[15]

Some early students in turn managed to unnerve their professors. Faculty members unfamiliar with frontier Texas mores and manners were shocked by some student practices. For instance, newly arrived from the ancient and cultured halls of Edinburgh, Professor William Keiller was astounded when medical students wore their cartridge belts to class. Although the students customarily unbuckled their belts and laid them on the benches at the beginning of class, it was just a matter of time before a dangerous fracas occurred. It happened in April 1895 when two male students got into an argument in the dissecting room of Old Red. The faculty minutes of April 27 reported the altercation climaxed with one of the students calling the other a "liar." In Texas frontier fashion, the offended party pulled out his pistol, fired—and thankfully missed. When the case went before a faculty disciplinary committee, not all the members viewed the incident in the same light. One committee member defended the shooter's behavior as that befitting a southern gentleman defending his honor. The majority, however, viewed it differently and, as a result, the offenders were "compelled to apologize to Dr. Keiller and the Faculty and be severely reprimanded by the Dean."[16] In another humorous, albeit less dangerous, instance, Howard Dudgeon (class of 1899) recalled seeing one of the Texans, "a big, burly freshman with pants tucked into the tops of his boots," slap the dignified Keiller resoundingly on the back at the conclusion of a lecture as he proclaimed, "Doc, you sure tell 'em. Don't you?"[17]

In the course of time, many UTMB students gained the respect and admiration of the medical school faculty. In his "Opening Address" to the Medical Department in 1903, Professor James E. Thompson extolled the perseverance and pluck demonstrated by early students in their efforts to acquire a solid medical education: "Students have been admitted with the poorest possible education, writing poor, crabbed and slow, spelling horrible. What the struggle the freshman year must have been to these Spartans can only be imagined. By sheer pertinacity they conquered.

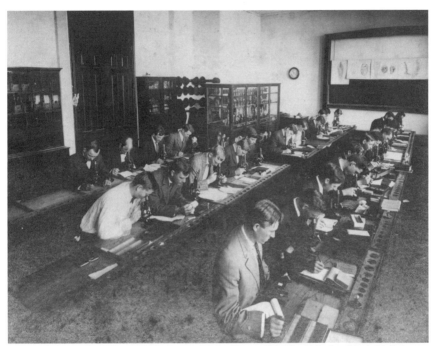

Pathology Lab, Old Red (1912). *Courtesy Blocker History of Medicine Collections, Moody Medical Library.*

We could see the evolution. Their writing became better, they expressed themselves more clearly because they were being taught to think clearly. They became more self-respecting and, at the end of the senior year, they were fresh men, entirely emancipated from all previous cramping habits of thought and action."[18] With a nod to these sentiments, Professor Allen J. Smith noted that one of the greatest sources of pride for the early faculty occurred when "Galveston graduates proved their worth by the highest grades" on the Texas licensure exams during the early 1900s.[19]

The issue of a poorly educated student body gradually diminished with the increase of academic standards. In 1910 the medical school began to require one year of college study for admission. However, it soon became apparent that even more college work was needed for the medical school's students to keep pace with the academic curriculum and for the school to maintain a highly respected reputation. By the fall of 1917, the credit requirement rose to two years of college and again to three years by 1937. The pharmacy school raised its standards far more slowly. For instance, when the medical school standards rose in 1917, the School of Pharmacy continued to welcome applicants who had completed only two years of high school. It was not until the fall of 1923 that entering freshmen were required to have a high school diploma.[20]

With the medical school's tightening of entrance requirements, more students arrived on campus better prepared to avoid the shame of flunking out. In 1910 Dean William Spencer Carter reported that the attrition rate had been reduced to 50 percent. Two years later, the rate had declined to one-third.[21] Nevertheless, the high-stress quest for academic survival remained a prominent feature of UTMB student culture for many years to come. The first day of class for Dr. Armond Goldman (class of 1953) during the fall of 1947 was just as traumatic as that of J. Gordon Bryson forty years before. Goldman remembered Professor Donald Duncan introduced the first year anatomy class thus: "Ladies and gentlemen, look around you. Next year many of the faces that you see today will not be here."[22] Goldman was tempted to quit immediately. And for good reason. From the 1920s through the 1960s, the medical school curriculum at UTMB was the one of the toughest in the nation. The Association of American Medical Colleges (AAMC) and the American Medical Association (AMA) recommended 4,000 curriculum hours over four years for graduation. UTMB professors required over 5,000 hours of study over the same time period. During the autumn of 1922, freshman Edith Bonnet (class of 1926) noted in her diary an anxiety-filled twenty-fifth birthday: "Tired, busy, worried, and ill with indigestion . . . This is a *hard* life." Three weeks later Bonnet's academic struggles had not dissipated. She wrote, "Failed in a Materia medica quiz and am doing very poorly in Anatomy and Chemistry. It's baffling to work so hard and get nowhere."[23] In 1932 a student revealed in the *University Medical* that the majority of his companions were frequent consumers of Tums, Bromo Seltzer, and aspirin, and, by the time they were seniors, they suffered from one or more of the following maladies: spastic colon, gastric neurosis, cirrhosis of the liver, hypertrophy of the heart, or cavitation of the lungs.[24] Although the course load eventually lightened, the four-year schedule remained intense.

Things got more heated when, at the beginning of World War II, the school implemented an accelerated physicians' training program that condensed the curriculum from four to three years. Male medical students experienced intense pressure from two directions: the travails brought on by an accelerated schedule and the knowledge that failure would likely send them into a war zone. Benjy F. Brooks (class of 1948) recalled the tension exhibited by some of her male classmates during the war years: "I can remember one man in my class went hysterically blind at the end of examinations. Another had anioneurotic edema and I can remember him taking his knife and cutting his socks as his ankles would swell . . .

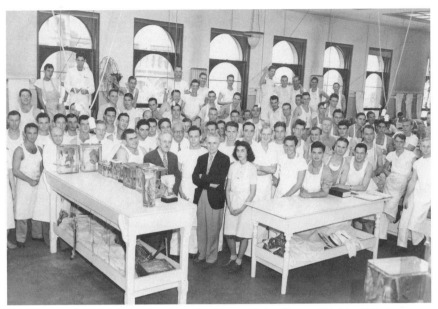

Freshman anatomy lab, Old Red (1943). *Courtesy Blocker History of Medicine Collections, Moody Medical Library.*

one had a bleeding ulcer, and I think that must have been some of the greatest tension that human beings could go through." If they flunked out, Brooks remembered, "We would get letters from them in three weeks and they would be medics on the front line."[25] Despite the return to a regular four-year schedule when the war ended, the School of Medicine remained tough with total class hours continuing to exceed the number recommended by the AAMC and AMA. The first two years of medical school remained a sprint, the junior year was heavy with lectures, and the seniors had a full year of clinical work.

The warm, muggy Gulf Coast climate did not help the situation. Long before air-conditioning arrived at Old Red and other campus buildings, students attended mandatory classes and labs in sometimes sweltering conditions. Chemistry professor Seth Mabry Morris recalled that in his early years of teaching at UTMB, lectures were given at two o'clock in the afternoon in the lower west lecture hall of Old Red. With no fans in the room, Morris admitted he "didn't blame the students for an occasional lapse into audible unconsciousness."[26] In 1923 the *University Medical* doffed its hat to any aspiring practitioner who steadfastly persevered in the face of heat, physical illness, and a grueling schedule. "We admit that the juggling artists are good—keeping several balls in the air at one time," observed the editor, "but a medical student kicking both feet to keep the mosquitoes away, one hand shooing the flies, and one hand mopping his brow while studying for examinations, has them all beat."[27] Little had changed when Bill Daeschner began his studies in 1942. Frequently, he reported, "the lecturer was just dripping when the hour was ended, and we'd sometimes have five or six hours of lecture in a row ... I don't think anybody heard anything the lecturer was saying. I'm not even sure the lecturer heard himself."[28]

Perhaps the greatest obstacles to obtaining a medical degree were reserved for female students. The fact that women wishing to study medicine were never officially denied admission to UTMB does not mean they were welcomed with open arms. Upholding the prevalent social prejudices of the day, certain members of the faculty and administration strongly objected to women entering the medical field. The first president of the University of Texas was one such individual. In 1896, Leslie Waggoner publicly expressed his sentiments in an address to the Texas Women's Press Association: "I understand that many young women are looking forward to studying medicine as a profession, and that already there is hardly a large city, even in the South, in which there are not one or two 'female doctors.' Against these personally I have not a word to say. But I deplore the effect of the example they set. The work of a doctor or surgeon is not the work for a woman. Because she is naturally a good nurse is no reason why she should cease to be the nurse and become the physician. We must have her watchful care, her tender sympathy, her anxious solicitude, but love must be the motive, not a fee."[29] Waggoner and the majority of late nineteenth-century society passionately believed the emancipation of women to compete and enter "men's" fields endangered the American family. The choice of a young female to enter the medical profession was considered a willful abandonment of her role as wife and mother.

In 1897, the year after Waggoner's speech to the press association, Marie Delalondre became the first female graduate of UTMB. Shortly afterwards, an admirer of Delalondre's trailblazing efforts, medical school Dean J. F.Y. Paine, made the following remarks to the Board of Regents: "While women have been admitted on equal terms with men to all the lectures and other exercises of both schools, medicine and pharmacy, since the organization of the Medical Department, it is worthy of mention that this is the first occasion on which they have been recommended for degrees. It is a source of gratification by the young lady made notably in the history of this college, by being the first of her gender to secure a degree in medicine is a modest and gentle lady, yet brave and independent."[30] In 1903 Minnie Fisher Cunningham became the first woman to graduate from the School of Pharmacy. Described by a journalist as "a 21-year-old ball of fire," Cunningham would eventually lead the women's suffragist movement in Texas. Despite the examples set by Delalondre and Cunningham, few young women matriculated at the medical and pharmacy schools. During the first fifty years, the percentage of female students at UTMB rarely extended beyond 5 percent of each entering class.[31]

A steel spine and a large dose of determination were vital attributes for young women wishing to pursue a medical degree at UTMB. Ruth Hartgraves (class of 1932) remembered on registration day, the school admissions officer told incoming students to form two lines: "those who really wanted to become doctors, and those who weren't quite sure." She said, "Some of the girls got into the second line, and then just walked right out the door . . . I wanted to be a doctor so bad I couldn't stand it, so I got in the first line."[32]

The decision to become a doctor was an extremely difficult one in a male-dominated world. Women whose professional ambitions took them out of the traditional female sphere often paid a price. Before Edith Bonnet left for medical school, a suitor informed her that he "wouldn't marry a woman that was a doctor."[33] His subsequent marriage to someone else painfully revealed to Edith that her choice of profession came at a price. On February 25, 1925, she wrote a soul-searching entry into her diary: "It makes me realize the finality of my deciding to study medicine . . . Since I am going to be a doctor I had better put *everything* I have into it; I've sacrificed so much to it that it would be extremely foolish to strain the gnats now. I do not know what I *should* have done. I do not know what I want to do."[34]

Once enrolled, young women studying medicine or pharmacy at UTMB often dealt with hostile male classmates who considered them intruders. The disapproval usually presented itself in the form of teasing, rude behavior, or vulgar remarks. "They teased me all the time," Sarah Rudnick Jourdin (class of 1918) admitted. "I think if I had been older I wouldn't have minded so much but it bothered me a lot . . . We would stand in the hallways [of Old Red] waiting for a class to begin . . . and I would find when I stuck my hand in the pocket of my sweater there would be a finger in there!"[35] As one of five female graduates out of a class of seventy-one, Dr. Margaret Magdeline Schoch (class of 1932) recalled being told she did not belong in medical school. "Many of them said to me," she related, "'I wouldn't let my wife practice medicine.'" Or, "Why are you doing all this? You know you are going to get married as soon as you get out of here and you are not going to use your profession."[36] In time, most female students often won over their antagonists and created lasting friendships. Years after she graduated, Edith Bonnet remained amused over

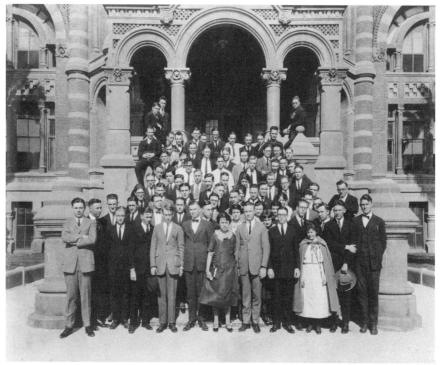

Freshman medical students, Old Red (1922). Edith Bonnet is standing in the front row, center. *Courtesy Blocker History of Medicine Collections, Moody Medical Library.*

the fact that some of her former persecutors became respected colleagues who referred patients to her—at times, their own children.[37]

As the twentieth century progressed, increasing numbers of female medical students darkened the doors of Old Red. A few were married when they arrived at UTMB and others married while students. In February 1938, third-year medical student, Virginia Levine married assistant professor of surgery Truman Blocker Jr. (class of 1933). The following December, Dr. Blocker gave birth to her first child, a son, missing only "a week or two of school" in the process. Grace Jameson (class of 1949) was married when she entered UTMB in 1945 and gave birth to her first child during her sophomore year. She missed only ten days of school and continued to nurse her baby after she returned to classes. Like Virginia Blocker, she recalled her classmates seemed to "cheer her on" through these events and took special interest in the new baby. Dr. Jameson later attributed her survival of motherhood and medical school to "the three H's: good health, good husband, and good [domestic] help."[38]

Far more daunting than the animosity of classmates was the censure by some of the male faculty. In an interview towards the end of her life, Edith Bonnet, who had entered medical school on scholarship, remembered an encounter with a faculty member who said it was needless for her to take the semester finals because he planned on seeing to it that she did not graduate. While Bonnet overcame that hurdle, she met a subsequent roadblock upon graduation in 1925. At that time, the hospital exercised a policy of accepting the nine top-ranking scholars of each graduating class. However, being male was one of the hospital requirements for interns. It took an appeal to Governor Miriam "Ma" Ferguson and unpleasant press coverage for John Sealy Hospital to remedy the situation. Bonnet and fellow scholar Frances Vanzant were provided contracts that made them the first female interns at John Sealy Hospital, "with the understanding that they would not be given certain courses applying to genito-urinary male patients."[39] Twenty-five years after Bonnet and Vanzant's struggle, Mary Ellen Haggard (class of 1951) experienced "sarcastic" remarks from a few male professors.[40]

Not all female medical and pharmacy students experienced the derision of male faculty members. Dr. Margaret Schoch "loved" all of her professors and did not experience any prejudicial stumbling blocks. Many male faculty were invaluable mentors to female students, including surgery professor Edgar Poth, who encouraged his student Benjy Brooks to go into pediatric surgery. In general, most women medical students seasoned themselves early on to the teasing and criticism of male students and some faculty. Like their compatriots at other coeducational medical schools in this period, female students labored to "blend in." They diligently studied, worked hard and, in so doing, formed meaningful relationships with the men.[41]

The presence of women professors at UTMB undoubtedly inspired many early female students. The first woman to serve on the medical school faculty was Marie Charlotte Schaefer. A 1900 graduate of the Medical Department, Dr. Schaefer joined the faculty after a year of postgraduate work at the University of Chicago and at Johns Hopkins University. After beginning her career as demonstrator of general biology, embryology, and histology, Schaefer was made a full professor of embryology in 1915, and in 1925 she became full professor of histology. As the only female in a field of male professors, Schaefer upheld a no-nonsense attitude at the medical school. William B. Sharp, a former chair of the department of bacteriology, remembered how students complained about Schaefer's high-level expectations. "She rode them hard!" Sharp recalled, "Where another teacher might ask them to describe a structure, Schaefer must have it in the minutest detail."[42] Dr. Schaefer did not have favorites. Female students remembered she was just as rigid and strict with the women in her class as the men.[43] Schaefer, who never married, also possessed a softer side. She took exceptional pride in the professional successes of her good students and endeavored to help those who were not so blessed. In the late spring of 1927, Dr. Schaefer died suddenly while conducting a laboratory session. She was fifty-three years old. Out of respect for Dr. Schaefer, all the May graduation parties and celebrations were canceled.[44]

By the time of Schaefer's death, other females had made their mark on the UTMB faculty. Violet Keiller (class of 1914), daughter of anatomy professor William Keiller, worked with James E. Thompson in surgical pathology until his death in 1927. Afterwards, she accepted a position of pathologist at Houston's Hermann Hospital before joining the faculty at the Baylor University Medical School when the institution moved from Dallas to Houston. Dr. Zidella Seibel Brener (class of 1935) remembered organic chemistry professor Marian Spencer Fay as a "fine teacher."[45] Others were part of husband-and-wife teams—both graduates of UTMB—who served on the faculty. These include Evangeline Ford (class of 1936); Virginia Blocker (class of 1939); Caroline Webster Rowe (class of 1944); Barbara Kolmen (class of 1957); and Lillian H. Lockhart (class of 1957).[46] Each played an important role in the training of new practitioners for the increasingly competitive field of medicine.

In some ways, the path for women enrolled in the school of nursing was smoother than that of their fellow females at the Medical Department. First, there were more of them. After it was incorporated into the University of Texas in 1896, the school grew rapidly with an eightfold enrollment increase over the next four decades. Between 1896 and 1941, over 3,000 young women had enrolled in the school. Second, nursing students endured less social pressure. By the late nineteenth century, nursing was not only viewed as a gender-appropriate profession, it was deemed essential to the dispensation of quality hospital care.[47]

Despite the positives, the nursing school environment was grueling. Students faced a daily routine that stressed discipline, self-sacrifice, and order. Pupil nurses worked twelve-hour shifts with built-in time for classwork and meals. The school of nursing curriculum, expanded in 1907 from two years to three, included a sequence of lectures by medical school faculty, demonstrations and "ward work." Nursing students attended classes in anatomy, physiology, pathology, materia medica, principles of nursing, surgical nursing, nursing of expectant women and children, emergency care, nutrition, administration of baths, physical therapy, and hygiene. Good health, strong backs, and sturdy feet were physical essentials, and the best student was "a keen learner but not too cocky; quick to respond, but not too aggressive, cheerful, but able to take her work seriously." Students

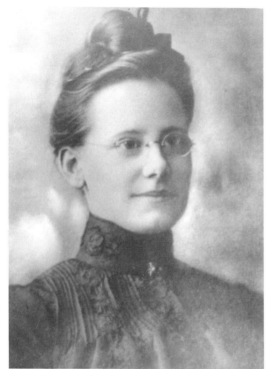

Left: Charlotte Marie Schaefer. The first woman to serve on the Medical Department faculty, Dr. Schaefer joined the staff in 1901 and served as chairman of the Department of Histology and Embryology from 1912 to 1927. *Courtesy Blocker History of Medicine Collections, Moody Medical Library.*

Below: Histology and embryology lab, Old Red (1912). Charlotte Schaefer can be seen in the background. *Courtesy Blocker History of Medicine Collections, Moody Medical Library.*

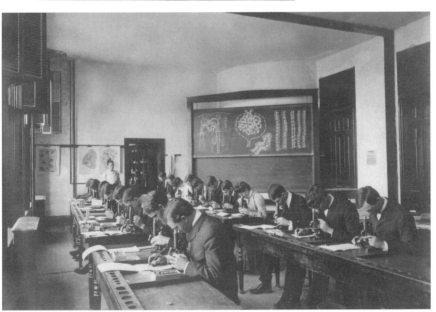

faced dismissal from the school if they were "unfit for the work," failed exams, or committed an infraction of the rules. Many found the atmosphere intolerable and withdrew from the program.[48]

The rigorous nursing school curriculum continued for the next several decades as the faculty enforced competitive guidelines. Beginning in 1935, the school limited applicants to those who had ranked in the upper half of their graduating high school class. In order to graduate, students were expected to pass all of their coursework and acquire a satisfactory rating on their work with patients. They became registered nurses (R.N.) once they passed the state board exam. The landscape changed considerably in 1946 when the UT regents approved the School of Nursing as a distinct unit from the University of Texas. The School of Medicine faculty no longer participated in the teaching of nursing students nor had a say in the nursing school curriculum. Nevertheless, the nursing students themselves remained a vital part of UTMB student culture.[49]

Despite the difficulties involved in achieving a degree from UTMB, student regard for the school and faculty was an important feature of the campus community. Recorded student memories of alumni provide evidence of the admiration and respect many students felt for their professors. In his school-day remembrances, Howard O. Smith (class of 1922) fondly described the faculty of his day. They included: "scholarly George H. Lee with his moustache and beard; Dr. Edward Randall, the Virginia gentleman who gently fingered his Phi Beta Kappa key while lecturing; Dr. James E. Thompson with his beautifully organized lectures, stiff bosom shirts and cuffs with links imported from England; Dr. A. O. Singleton with his humorous remarks, occasionally cutting, but always truthful."[50] In his "Recollections," Howard Dudgeon reminisced about the captivating lectures of William Keiller, who entranced students with magnificent chalkboard illustrations, charts, and "splendidly mounted and beautifully prepared specimens," all created by his own artistic hands. Short, slight, and bald, Keiller regularly greeted new students with "Hello Freshmen!" in his high-pitched voice.[51] The customary welcome issued by Keiller's successor, Harry O. Knight, was another highlight. Each autumn, Knight urged the freshmen: "You've got to stand on your own bottoms and let the chips fall where they may."[52] One alumnus who graduated in 1953 remembered a pet dog attending the anatomy lectures of Raymond Blount ("a very nice mad man") in the Old Red amphitheater. This canine undoubtedly witnessed Blount's habit of throwing an eraser with "unerring aim" at any student caught not paying attention in class.[53]

The assigning of nicknames to faculty was another means of expressing regard. "All of the faculty had some kind of a nickname," wrote Howard O. Smith, "which was really complimentary even though it might not have sounded so at the time, especially to the individual so named."[54] The chairman of the biochemistry department, Byron Hendrix, was "Lumpy Jaw" because of a facial nerve paralysis. One of his successors, the red-headed Andrew Ormsby, was the "Red Fox." The brusque demeanor of Professor of Medicine Raymond Gregory earned him the nickname of "Tiger." Nurses labeled James Thompson "old Hellfire and Damnation" for the surgery chair's flagrant use of profanity in the operating room. Some faculty earned nicknames according to the opposite of what they were: for instance, the distinguished professor of anatomy, William "Wild Bill" Keiller, or the characteristically dour professor of surgery, Edgar "Smiley" Poth. One of the most colorful and beloved of the early professors was Seth Mabry Morris. Fondly nicknamed "Old Test Tube" by his students, the chemistry professor possessed an eccentric albeit frustrating classroom habit of writing chemical equations on the blackboard with his right hand while simultaneously erasing them with his left. Morris also reportedly frightened many Galveston residents when he drove around town as the owner of the first automobile on the Island—a 1902 Oldsmobile.[55]

The student practice of honoring faculty members with nicknames extended to their most cherished campus building. It was during this era of assigning nicknames that students began affectionately calling what was formerly labeled the "Medical Department Building" or "the red building" as "Old Red." For years to come, the characteristics of everyday life within Old Red became the stuff of treasured memories: the boisterous class bell that rang so loudly it woke students sleeping in off-campus housing; the great rush between classes to access via an intricate passageway the only available restroom in the building; laboratory towel fights; and long hours of taking class notes in open-windowed rooms while beautiful white oleanders bloomed below. The omnipresent flocks of pigeons provided additional interest. As a medical student during the early 1950s, Armond Goldman purposely occupied a seat on the north side of the amphitheater during warm weather "so I could not only hear and see the presentations from the lecturers but also witness the daily flights of pigeons that came through the large open windows that face the south." On occasion, Goldman recalled, "these avian creatures innocently bombarded a lecturer or student, but in the main they (the birds that is) were well behaved and remained on the outskirts of the lecture hall."[56] Regardless of the era, student affinity for Old Red was based upon traditional pride, inspiration, and sentimental charm.

Although academic studies were the central focus at UTMB, students still managed to carve out time for fun. With Old Red as a backdrop, remarkable initiative was displayed in creating a dynamic student com-

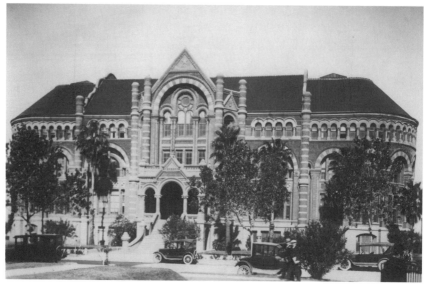

Daily scene in front of Old Red (1920s). *Courtesy Rosenberg Library.*

munity. Beginning with the first decade, medical and pharmacy students organized a dining club, a vibrant student council, and the *University Medical* journal; participated in athletic groups, and singing competition; and, for a short time, supported a college orchestra. To entertain themselves, students staged theatrical productions, traveled to horse shows and UT football games, hosted clambakes and dances, attended beach parties, and enjoyed other local Galveston attractions. Taking a date for a casual stroll along the Galveston seawall was a very popular pastime during the 1910s and early 1920s. The "seawall brigade," as it was called in the *University Medical*, and going to local dance halls and clubs were courtship activities that appealed to even the poorest medical student. The social highlight of the year was the Final Ball for seniors, a formal dinner and dance held in one of the local hotel ballrooms.[57]

A highly popular diversion for the students during the first twenty-five years was class competitions. During these years, when fewer students possessed a college background, spirited class rivalries were central to life within its walls. Never having experienced undergraduate life, they sought to recreate nineteenth-century college traditions at their professional school. Moreover, this form of class bonding helped serve the social and psychological needs of students who, perhaps for the first time, found themselves miles from home. Classes typically organized with class officers, class mottos, class colors, and creative class yells. In 1902 the freshman medical class adopted class hats sporting their colors, blue and orange.[58]

Class yells often made it into the University of Texas yearbook, the *Cactus*. The chosen cheer for the Pharmacy Class of 1901 went as follows:

Sulphur, Borax, NH3
Cline, Milburn, T. C. P.,
Ipecac, Opium, Tansy tea,
Senior Class of Pharmacy![59]

The medical class of 1909 went several steps further with this audacious ballad:

Well man, sick man, dead man, stiff.
Cut 'em up, Cut 'em up; what's the diff.
Bloody bones, Bloody bones, Sis Boom Ba,
Texas Medics, Rah! Rah! Rah![60]

Perhaps the most passionate expressions of undergraduate fellowship occurred between freshmen and sophomores, or at times, between the freshmen and the rest of the student body. The freshman "rush" was a favorite pastime during the fall term. This activity entailed one group of students shoving or "rushing" another as they attempted to depart en masse from a particular location, for example, Allen J. Smith's pathology lecture. The jostling and shoving often continued until a fight broke out. Often by the end of the skirmish, at least one hapless freshman found himself at the bottom of the steps of Old Red. In a 1905 issue of *University Medical*, a sophomore alluded to the physical and ego-bruising effects of this custom: "The Sophomores hope that, by free and continuous application of the rod, they may help the Freshman child from becoming spoiled."[61] Often unwilling to take such abuse lying down, freshman class members struck back and sometimes won. A victory in October 1902 was commemorated with a verse sung to the tune of "Sing a Song of Sixpence":

Sing a song of broken bones and sadly tethered vesture,
Eight and forty sophomores coming from a lecture.
The mighty freshmen rushed them and they began to squeal,
They suddenly dropped their notebooks
And took to the heel.
Chorus:
When the rush is over you ought to hear them cry,
Please, Oh, Please, Dear Freshman,

Won't you let us by?
Then the noble freshmen follow with a yell,
What they do to sophs wouldn't do to tell.
Let others take the warning, don't think yourselves too wise,
For the freshmen of naughty '03 will rush you to the skies![62]

The lack of enthusiasm by the female students for this exclusively male practice can only be imagined. In any case, by 1912, the class rush had become a tradition of the past. The class rushes during the fall of 1911 were so disruptive that Dean William Spencer Carter demanded their abolishment. The timing was right. By the time of Carter's announcement, many students were entering UTMB having already tasted the absurd merriment of the undergraduate world. By 1911, at least a third of the incoming freshmen class possessed a college degree. Few had the desire to repeat undergraduate antics in medical school. "[We] have been to college before," one freshman contemptuously noted in the *University Medical*, "and strange to say, the ideas we have brought from there do not include throwing the new men down a flight of stone stairs, so that the interns at the hospital might practice on setting their bones, nor even tearing up the clothes and trampling the watches of the fellows who have to scratch to make their way through school . . . when the next year's Freshmen come in, we intend to offer them the glad hand of welcome, and to do our best to imbue them with that spirit which is putting our school into the front rank among institutions of its kind." While future freshman classes continued to receive a sizable dose of teasing, their relationship with upperclassmen, especially sophomores, became decidedly more congenial.[63]

Fraternities were another extremely popular aspect of the student community at UTMB. They provided room and board, companionship and psychological support, and built-in study groups. Fraternity groups sponsored intramural sports contests and hosted numerous parties—some rather raucous. They also provided an avenue for students and faculty to socialize outside the classroom. The first fraternities, the Sigma Ribbon Society and the Jolly Bone Jugglers, were organized in 1896 as local groups without a national affiliation. The Jolly Bone Jugglers were founded specifically as to provide diversion from the daily pressures of medical school. Charter members claimed that although "gleeful recreation is not altogether forbidden," the primary objective of the club was to give members of the different medical school classes an opportunity to become better acquainted and promote "a feeling of universal brotherhood" among the members. The president was labeled the "Giant Skeleton." Other officers were titled Grand Mongul, Bone Box, Three-Eyed Monster, Phantom

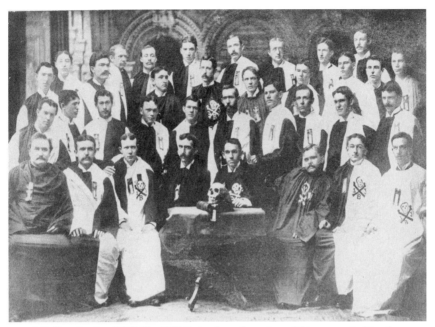

Jolly Bone Jugglers (1898). The 1898 *Cactus* pictured members of this group attired in robes embellished with skull and crossbones. *Courtesy Blocker History of Medicine Collections, Moody Medical Library.*

Hand, and Bony Warrior.[64] A photo in the 1898 *Cactus* pictures the light-hearted group wearing robes decorated with skull and crossbones.

Eventually, both the Jolly Bone Jugglers and the Sigma Ribbon Society dissolved in favor of nationally affiliated fraternities. By 1916 seven national fraternity chapters were active at UTMB. In 1914 delegates from the oldest and largest fraternities—Phi Chi, Alpha Kappa Kappa, Phi Beta Pi, and Phi Alpha Sigma—established the group Osteon, known primarily for hosting the highly popular Final Ball for seniors. Later reorganized as the Osteon Costume Ball, this affair adorned the social calendars of local debutantes and premed students from around the state. By 1924 the groups Kappa Psi, Beta Phi Sigma, and Phi Delta Epsilon, a national Jewish fraternity, had also joined the string of UTMB fraternities. In 1922 female medical students organized the only sorority at UTMB: the Texas Rho chapter of Alpha Epsilon Iota, a group that attracted most of the female medical students through the 1930s.[65]

The fraternity and sorority presence at UTMB differed from that found at undergraduate colleges and universities. Rather than representing only elite or affluent members of the student body, the Greek organizations at UTMB included most, and, in some years, virtually all the students. During the 1923 school year, 245 male medical students—an astounding 99.5 percent of those enrolled—belonged to a fraternity. Similarly, 98 percent of male students were fraternity members in 1944, almost 95 percent in 1954, and 96.8 percent in 1966. Although in 1922 Alpha Epsilon Iota sorority was founded with only five members, by 1939 the group claimed 31 of the 34 female medical students at UTMB. Judging from these statistics, it is possible to conclude that students not affiliated with a Greek organization did so by choice. Overt exclusionary practices were not apparent until the early 1950s and 1960s when the first African American students were barred from joining the organizations.[66]

One of the highlights of fraternity and sorority life was Rush Week. In their vigorous competition for members, fraternities hosted a dizzying series of meetings, fetes, and dinners. During the automobile craze of the 1920s, freshman Felix Butte wrote his girlfriend: "The Phi Chis met me at the train Wednesday in a big Pierce Arrow with a chauffeur, then later took me out in a Lincoln. I rode in all kinds of cars till I pledged."[67] Medical pioneer Mavis Kelsey pledged Alpha Kappa Kappa in the mid-1930s. "Our annual initiation party was an important event," Kelsey recalled, "Home brew, made in the fraternity house, was served. There was a continuous open bar . . . There were beach parties and softball games. Some upperclassmen went to Sui Jen to gamble, and a group walked through the red light district at night."[68] Compared to the "class rush," fraternity rushes were genteel affairs. But the same could not be said for the fraternity initiation—the real heir to the intimidating class rush. A reporter from the *University Medical* wrote in 1924: "We pray that these four highly esteemed freshmen (Phi Delta Chi pledges) live through their initiation—you know the vats in the stiff room are already crowded."[69] Another writer quipped to the 1927 Beta Phi Sigma pledges that after their initiation, the "lecture rooms will be provided with cushions the following week."[70] The situation was little better for female sorority pledges. During the 1920s and 1930s, Alpha Epsilon Iota members put their initiates through a series of harassments that included attending class on crutches, with their arms and legs bandaged, or wearing foul-smelling anatomy aprons as they consumed "autopsy meat" (roast beef) and "boils in pus" (creamed onions) with dissecting instruments for silverware.[71]

Chapter houses provided each fraternity with an energetic base of operations. Before 1941, these rented or purchased old Victorian mansions in Galveston's east end served as living quarters, study hall, and primary social outlet. Some of the houses had large sleeping porches where many members slept, especially in warm weather. Between 1941 and 1966, all of the UTMB medical fraternities moved out of their old mansions into new houses of modern design. Many fraternity houses held frequent "bull sessions" where members discussed the medical field, their families, sweethearts, personal dreams, and goals. Fraternity mates also assembled for study sessions and used files of old quizzes to prepare for exams.[72]

Wild parties and uninhibited alcohol consumption were a matter of course at many fraternity chapter houses. C. M. Phillips (class of 1931) recalled that each fraternity hosted an annual dance. In preparation for the big event, large supplies of bootleg liquor bottled in nearby Dickinson would be delivered to the fraternity house.[73] During the 1940s, the Phi Chis were known for their lively toga parties and the Phi Betas annually hosted a Hawaiian luau complete with grass skirts, flowered shirts, and leis. According to UTMB Professor of Surgery Jay Collie Fish (class of 1958), the traditional beverage for the Phi Beta event was a punch laced with grain alcohol procured undercover from John Sealy Hospital.[74] Some faculty balked over the fraternity-hosted escapades. Dr. John Sinclair was known to sternly reprimand Osteon inductees who trudged into class after a spirited evening with fraternity brothers, still dressed in their tuxedos, the Osteon pledge uniform. Virginia Irvine Blocker (class of 1939) remembered that Professor of Medicine George R. Hermann used to recite in class the number of bottles he found in his alley after an Alpha Kappa Kappa party.[75]

Occasionally, fraternity affairs got out of hand, compelling the UTMB administration to intervene. In the early 1920s, the college banned Theta Nu Epsilon fraternity because it had become infamous for "enthusiastic banquets" and "bizarre entertainments."[76] In the late 1920s, two young men accepted to UTMB from Rice University were denied admission into the medical school after attending a Phi Beta Pi dance with "dates" acquired from Galveston's red light district.[77] The "Osteon Affair" of 1939 was the most notorious fraternity infraction during these years. A series of fights erupted between visiting Rice football players and medical students during the annual Osteon costume dance. The foray climaxed when the daughter of a prominent faculty member received an unintentional smack in the jaw. The result included a visit from local police, complaints from irate mothers, and a severe threat from the medical school administration to abolish the intra-fraternity group. A compromise between students and administration to make the ball a more "formal" affair saved the event from swift extinction.[78]

In general, UTMB administration and faculty were tolerant, even supportive of fraternity activities. Many of the faculty had joined fraternities during their student days, and a few were charter members. Moreover, an important advantage of fraternities involved the opportunity for faculty and alumni to create close relationships with the students. One such mentor was Texas Medical Center founder Ernst William Bertner (class of 1911), a charter member of the Alpha Kappa Kappa (AKK) fraternity. Considered "one of the boys," few fraternity activities were off limits for the ever-popular Bertner—including the accompaniment of young AKK's in a spirited jaunt through the red light district during Rush Week. Bertner and other AKK's returned annually to join in the fun, inspire, and share advice regarding internships.

In his autobiography, Mavis Kelsey, an AKK pledge in the mid-1930s, recalled a time when Bertner's influence was especially valued. By 1935, the Great Depression had tossed the AKK chapter into a sea of red ink. "The grocery bill alone was $1,000 a month," wrote Kelsey, "about the same as the total monthly dues. The local Gengler's Grocery, the utilities, the phone company, and numerous other creditors were about to shut us down."[79] The fraternity came in grave danger of losing their chapter house, the old Suderman home located on 14th Street and Avenue E. Coming to the rescue, Bertner organized an effort to retain the AKK chapter house through generous contributions by fellow fraternity alumni. The endeavor worked, but the bailout came with conditions. Bertner kept the fraternity on a strict budget, personally doling out select amounts of money until the financial crisis had passed. The fraternity remained grateful for years afterward. Heart specialist Denton Cooley remembered when he pledged AKK in the early 1940s Bertner was considered the "patron saint" of the fraternity.[80] The Suderman home remained the AKK chapter house until 1966, when the fraternity moved into a modern thirty-eight-bed residence "complete with color TV and a swimming pool."[81]

Female Greek members did not enjoy the same advantages as their male counterparts. For instance, Alpha Epsilon Iota sorority did not have a chapter house. Its membership resided at University Hall or rooming houses located near campus. They did not have access to quiz files for exams or experience close bonds with female alumni. They also rarely entertained. Medical and pharmacy women sometimes gave "teas," or attended those given by women in the Galveston community. As a result, female medical students did not have access to the same traditions and connections that male students had. Friendships with other fellow female students were related more to living arrangements or work situations than sorority affiliation.[82]

Nursing students fared better in terms of housing and social life. In 1932, still living separately from the medical student population, student nurses experienced the pleasure of moving into a lavish new residence hall. The second Rebecca Sealy Nurses' Residence—a four-story, richly decorated facility that accommodated one hundred and sixty students—

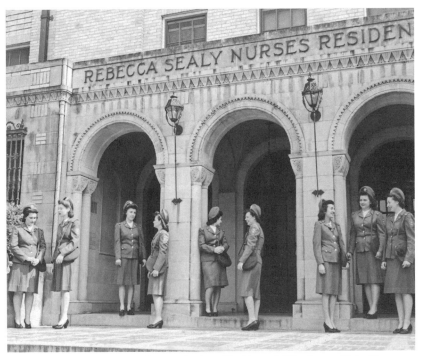

School of Nursing Cadets, Rebecca Sealy Nurses' Residence (1946). *Courtesy Blocker History of Medicine Collections, Moody Medical Library.*

sported a red-tiled roof, red–and–brown tiled foyer floor, carved walnut chairs and benches with leather backs, and a fireplace with a seal of the University of Texas carved into its stone mantel. In addition to bedrooms and bathrooms, the building contained a living room, library, reception room, auditorium, diet laboratory, classrooms, offices for teachers, a small infirmary, and patio gardens. The nurses' home served as the primary student residence until 1955 when several new and air-conditioned dormitories were opened at UTMB including Morgan and Vinsant Halls.[83]

Dormitory life was highly important to nursing students. The dorms were for these young women the equivalent of chapter houses for male medical students. Students of all classes often benefited from the academic encouragement dormitory life provided. Junior students coached the freshmen and sophomores through their basic science courses. Seniors helped juniors in their first year of clinical work in the hospital. Nurses also enjoyed an active social life. Like fraternity houses, each dormitory had its own informal initiation rites including, for instance, the time-honored duty of first-year students of scrubbing front steps with toothbrushes.[84]

Student nurses were also enthusiastic hostesses and gave more parties than any other single group at UTMB. They threw entertainments for interns and freshmen, to celebrate Halloween, Valentine's Day, and Christmas, hosted a variety of dances, and established a tradition of an annual talent show for the student body. The beautifully furnished living room of the second Rebecca Sealy Nurses' Residence was as much a meeting place for UTMB students as any of the fraternity houses. For a time, it was regarded as "the only decent gathering place" on campus for social activities among students. In 1948 the Sealy and Smith Foundation contributed $4,000 to refurnish the lounge of the residence. In contrast to many women students in the medical school, student nurses openly expressed their interest in dating medical students. Judging from the numerous comments in the *University Medical* regarding "nursitis" or "Nurseville," the male medical students reciprocated these sentiments. In the early 1940s, the nursing students' column in the *University Medical* rarely missed an opportunity to comment on the "cute" new students or even upon the desire of many nursing students to marry doctors. During the war years, the nursing students warned the medics that the many soldiers in town presented serious competition for the nursing students' attention. Yet, even though the nursing students enjoyed dating and having a good time, they were also industrious and hardworking, and therefore found it important to maintain a social identity apart from medical and pharmacy students.[85]

In general, UTMB students socialized separately from the larger Galveston community. This was due, in part, to the distasteful opinion locals held of male medical students. Galvestonians often deemed the students as a rowdy, disreputable bunch—a viewpoint undoubtedly enhanced by some wild parties and antics. Although many students did not fit the unsavory mold created by detractors, the reputation stuck for several decades. The town-versus-gown relationship began to improve in the 1920s. Aware of their bad name in the community, many UTMB students began to attend local churches and synagogues and participate more fully in the Island activities and culture. Moreover, as the social position of physicians improved, the more kindly disposed Galveston's upper classes became toward the UTMB student body. Male students escorted local debutantes to prestigious events, including the much-celebrated annual Artillery Ball.[86]

Demographic changes following World War II further modified the student culture of UTMB. The "G.I. Bill of Rights" passed by the United States Congress in 1944, provided educational benefits to World War II veterans. Those who chose medical school were significantly older, more mature and sophisticated than the usual fresh-out-of-college medical student. Many veterans were married—a fact that contributed to a growing

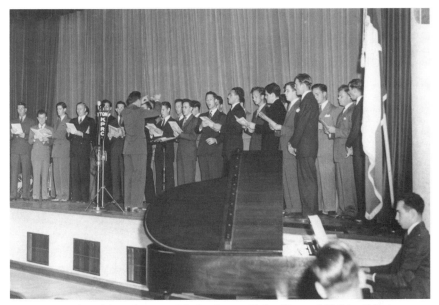

UTMB Glee Club performance (1941). *Courtesy Blocker History of Medicine Collections, Moody Medical Library.*

and irreversible trend. Throughout the late 1940s and early 1950s, the portion of married students varied from one-tenth to one-half. By 1961 at least 30 percent of the medical students were married.[87] These focused and committed veterans and their spouses (mostly wives) contributed to a more serious atmosphere at the UTMB campus.

Despite the extreme disparity in age and life experiences between the veterans and the younger students, the two groups did not isolate themselves from each other. Veterans joined the fraternities, and most of the single ones lived in the fraternity houses. Although the wild fraternity parties and hijinks continued through the early 1960s, married men, especially those with children, had less time for much drinking with their classmates. Still, fraternity-sponsored activities remained at the center of social life at UTMB. Parties and dances highlighted the social calendars of both singles and married couples. Sunday dinner was a big tradition at the Phi Chi house where fraternity members, their families, and alumni gathered before the beginning of another rigorous school week. All manner of intramural sports contests also remained popular. Jay Collie Fish remembers that each chapter house during the 1950s had a ping-pong table, and bridge tournaments were held in the basement of Old Red.[88]

The postwar student body experienced other important changes, including an increasingly diverse student body. Between 1900 and 1940, a few students with Hispanic surnames graduated from UTMB. Emma Domingo (class of 1900) was the first to graduate from the School of Pharmacy, followed by Alfonzo Y. García in 1908. Daniel Saenz (class of 1921) paved the way for other Hispanics in the School of Medicine, and in 1926 Simona López was the first Hispanic to graduate from the School of Nursing. More Hispanics were admitted after 1960. The medical school's first two Asian graduates, Mitsuharu Hoshino of Japan and Ho-Sheng Huang of South China, finished in 1920.[89] African American admission began with Herman Barnett (class of 1953), a World War II fighter pilot in 1949. Enrolled via a contract with Texas Southern University in Houston, Barnett was expected to stay at UTMB until a medical school opened at TSU. The Texas Legislature had appropriated money in 1949 for a "Negro medical school," but the institution never materialized. Barnett was officially enrolled in 1950.[90]

Although Herman Barnett's presence on the UTMB campus initially caused a stir, he was soon recognized as a truly outstanding student who earned considerable respect from both classmates and professors. Fellow classmate Armond Goldman remembers Barnett was the only student who could be suddenly called upon to recite in Professor Raymond Blount's anatomy class and not "mess up."[91] When Barnett graduated in 1953, only 2 percent of the nation's physicians were African American. Barnett's female counterpart was Virginia Stull, who in 1966 became the first black woman to receive a medical degree from UMTB. The nursing school began admitting black applicants in 1957, even though the numbers remained small for several years. Wilina Iona Gatson became the first black student to earn a nursing degree in 1960.[92]

These early black students, however, were not included in the regular campus social life. Their housing was separate from white students, and they were encouraged to form their own student organizations. Fraternity organizations were closed to blacks. Gatson, on the other hand, received considerable support from her fellow students nurses, including bringing her take-out food back from local restaurants that did not serve blacks. In general, however, UTMB smoothly rode the winds of change. Between 1949 and 1975, fifty-seven blacks enrolled in the School of Medicine. By the end of that period, thirty African Americans had earned their medical degrees. A few joined fraternities after they integrated in 1968. Throughout future decades, UTMB strove to maintain a racial and ethnically inclusive environment for its students. By 2009, one-third of the graduates belonged to minority groups—a proportion larger than any other medical school in the state.[93]

From first-day jitters and burning the midnight oil to a potpourri of extracurricular activities, a vibrant student culture existed at UTMB that involved everyone. Although the subcultures of school, class, gender, and, in later years, race played an important role in their medical school experience, there was much that bound students together. Each student—whether male or female—sought a career in medicine. As professionals, they would care for the sick and work to advance the medical profession in their communities. And most—when they had the time to do so—would fondly remember their lives as students within the halls of Old Red.

Chapter 5
RESTORING A LEGACY

IT PROBABLY NEVER OCCURRED to most of those who worked, studied, and sometimes played inside Old Red that one day the building might be gone. But such a possibility became a genuine threat as UTMB advanced into a world in which many historical structures were slowly becoming obsolete. The task of preserving Old Red became a formidable one, requiring years of effort by a vast array of determined and talented individuals. However, the results of this impressive campaign to save Old Red and its subsequent renovation continue to thrill and delight the beholder.

UTMB changed dramatically in the postwar decades. Having withstood the turbulence of the Spies era and World War II, massive storms, and a manmade disaster in Texas City, the school turned its energy toward academic growth and development. As chief administrative officer, Chauncey Leake fiercely promoted UTMB as an institution of national and international renown. With the encouragement of Leake and his successor, Truman G. Blocker Jr., UTMB faculty in the 1940s, 1950s, and 1960s assumed more large-scale research projects than ever before. Donald Duncan, George William Eggers, Ardroozny Packchanian, Morris Pollard, and other professors utilized federal and private dollars to conduct biomedical research. Between 1946 and 1966, UTMB faculty received $10 million in research grants from the United States Public Health Service alone. The training of physicians, nurses, and other health care professionals was also central to its postwar mission. The school experienced a dramatic growth in doctoral and master's degree programs that culminated in 1973 with the establishment of a separate Graduate School of the Biomedical Sciences.[1]

Burgeoning research and teaching programs required greater classroom space and technologically refined research facilities. In support of these initiatives, UTMB added to its campus the Gail Borden Laboratory Building (1952), the Surgical Research Laboratories (1964), the Libbie Moody Thompson Basic Sciences Building (1971), and the Moody

Medical Library (1972). Aided by state, federal, and private funds, UTMB expanded its care of the sick. It added a new John Sealy Hospital (1954), a new Children's Hospital (1978), the Jennie Sealy Hospital (1968), the Shriners Burns Institute (1966), and facilities for ambulatory care (1966). The medical school increasingly took on a new look.[2]

Throughout the 1950s and 1960s, Old Red, now officially named the Ashbel Smith Building, continued to function much as it always had. Students attended lectures and demonstrations in classrooms and the east amphitheater, freshmen dissected cadavers in the anatomy laboratory on the third floor, and staff occupied office space. For many years, the basement of Old Red served as a popular "hang-out" for students. According to alumnus Jay Collie Fish (class of 1958) bridge tournaments and other recreational activities were favorite pastimes, especially for the many students who lacked the luxury of a car or television set. Popular bridge tournaments and other recreational activities were held on a regular basis.[3]

Still, time and Mother Nature took a heavy toll on Old Red. As UTMB expanded, academic activity and resources began to stream away from its institutional heart. Sophisticated technology requirements rendered many of Old Red's spaces obsolete. As classrooms and laboratories moved to sleeker, more specialized buildings, Old Red increasingly became a space for auxiliary services. Over time, the structure's once vital interior was downgraded to house the school bookstore, a postal substation, and repair shops. Changing needs over the years led to extensive remodeling of the interior. Dropped ceilings were installed to cover mechanical systems. The original stately classroom and laboratory spaces were sectioned off for office and storage. The grand lecture room-amphitheater on the west end of the building was removed and the third floor extended into the void. Maintenance to the building became segmented, attendant only to the needs of particular pockets of space.[4]

The exterior of Old Red also began showing considerable wear and tear. The natural elements and alterations to the exterior began to whittle away at the original character of the building. Decades of storms and harsh, corrosive sea winds marred its beautiful facade. Fire escapes installed on the exterior diminished the structure's visual elegance. In time, boarded windows, missing panes, cracks in the masonry, weeds sprouting through large cracks in the masonry, and tiles absent from the roof affirmed structural neglect and decay.[5]

In 1961 Hurricane Carla, the largest hurricane of record in Texas, struck the Island with wind gusts of up to 175 miles per hour. Coming ashore at Port O'Connor, the massive storm and ensuing tornado wiped a rugged swath of destruction across Galveston, killing or injuring dozens of individuals and demolishing more than 100 structures. While John Sealy

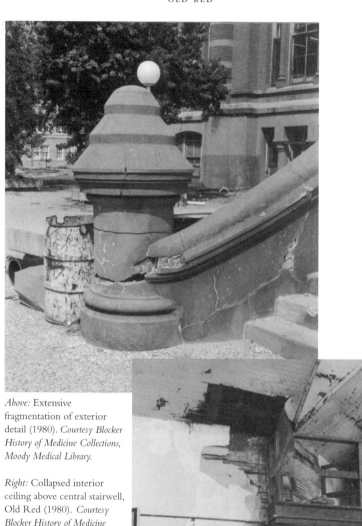

Above: Extensive
fragmentation of exterior
detail (1980). *Courtesy Blocker
History of Medicine Collections,
Moody Medical Library.*

Right: Collapsed interior
ceiling above central stairwell,
Old Red (1980). *Courtesy
Blocker History of Medicine
Collections, Moody Medical
Library.*

Hospital served as the city's most populous shelter, housing and feeding an estimated 3,000 evacuees, Old Red withstood the storm alone, its personnel evacuated from the building. Both Old Red and John Sealy endured flooding and considerable damage to their exteriors. However, when it came to repairs, Old Red, now deemed far less important, received minimal attention.[6]

Hurricane Carla dealt Old Red another devastating blow. In the storm's aftermath, UTMB officials displayed little concern or interest in keeping the old medical school building around. Instead, they proposed a demolition. The plan involved improving the condition of Old Red to keep it usable until 1969 when the building would be torn down to allow space for new campus structures. When word spread that Old Red was destined for the wrecking ball, an outcry arose among the UTMB community and Galveston. "Rumors that the old building is to be demolished to give way to more modern and more necessary projects to serve the needs of the medical center create a tinge of sadness," *Galveston Daily News* reporter Lillian Herz poignantly wrote in 1962, "not only because we love the old buildings which are traditional here and which form a part of the city's historical past, but because we personally recall many pleasant memories – of climbing the old stairways, of visiting laboratories, of chatting with old friends who were the backbone of the medical profession here in the old brick building . . . when the time comes and the building is demolished, it will leave a void in Galveston difficult to fill, and a feeling of regret in many alumni."[7]

The news concerning Old Red came at a fortuitous time, for it coincided with the rise of the historical preservation movement in Galveston. The tourism industry on the Island had changed in the postwar period. Although vacationers traveled to Galveston to enjoy the beaches, seafood, and other recreational venues, they also were increasingly drawn to another unique aspect of the Island: its architectural past. The city had grown slowly in the decades following the 1900 storm. As a consequence, a multitude of Victorian-era structures, many designed by Nicholas Clayton, remained extant, deteriorating casualties of time. In addition to Old Red, other derelict structures in Galveston included the Grand Opera House, the old City National Bank Building, and the Garten Verein Pavilion. By the late 1950s, Galveston citizens began to take stock of local architectural relics and their relevance to the Island's distinctive character and identity. "Like old persons reflecting upon their lives in order to understand them," writes historian David McComb, "Galvestonians began to consider and value history."[8] In the most pragmatic sense, preservation of historic island buildings meant profits for the city.[9]

In 1957 members of the Galveston elite established the Galveston Historical Foundation (GHF) to spearhead the preservation of one of the oldest surviving structures on the Island, the Williams-Tucker House. The effort was successful, and the home began welcoming visitors in 1959. Four years later, the Clayton-designed "Bishop's Palace" opened its doors to tourists. However, the goal of GHF went beyond mere structural preservation. While each building was restored on the outside, the interiors were adapted to current community needs. This concept of adaptive restoration encouraged a multiplicity of uses—from shops to restaurants, to office and apartment space. In this manner, the buildings would survive to serve the Galveston community and its many visitors.[10] At its peak, the historic preservation movement in Galveston resulted in the creation of the East End Historical District, the Silk Stocking National Historic District, the restoration of the Grand Opera House, the 1861 Custom House, and many other architectural gems.[11]

As one of Nicholas Clayton's finest structures, Old Red received historical recognition from a variety of sources. In 1962 the Texas State Historical Survey (now known as the Texas Historical Commission) officially recognized Old Red and ten other Galveston buildings as Texas Historical Landmarks. The honor was noted with a Texas State Historical Survey medallion attached to the side of each structure. Encouraged by the public's support of these landmarks, the GHF conducted a detailed survey of twenty-five buildings highlighting the historical and architectural significance of each. Old Red topped the list that included the James M. Brown House (or Ashton Villa), Open Gates, the George Sealy Mansion, and buildings along the Strand. In 1969 Old Red was selected for the National Register of Historic Places. The cradle of Texas medical education, Old Red was acknowledged as one of three extant nineteenth century buildings in the United States that at one time housed an entire medical school.[12] In November, Texas Lieutenant Governor Ben Barnes and UT System Chair Frank C. Erwin joined UTMB President Truman G. Blocker in a ceremony whereby Old Red received two official Texas State Historical Survey markers: one for the site of the original medical college and one for the historic building itself.[13]

Surprisingly, despite the receipt of national and state honors, Old Red remained on the endangered list at UTMB. Without a plan to preserve it, Old Red continued to deteriorate throughout the decade following Hurricane Carla. While faculty continued to give lectures in some classrooms and laboratories, the majestic medical college building served UTMB primarily as storage space. A member of the class of 1969, UTMB Department of Surgery chair Courtney M. Townsend remembered Old Red as "an old, not well kept up space." The back stair provided the only access to the building, and, "the amphitheater had several windows out and "Pigeons were in there all the time."[14] In 1971, with the intent to promote campus development, the UT regents proposed to replace Old Red with a parking lot. The decade-long reprieve for Old Red was drawing to a close.

The slated demise of Old Red distressed many UTMB students, employees, and alumni. Many agreed with Galveston County Judge Ray Holbrook, who equated the destruction of the landmark to "selling the medical school down the river." For UTMB alumni and many other Texas citizens, Old Red symbolized the genesis of an impressive medical program, one that developed from a small school into a major educational, research, and referral center. Thousands of physicians and other health specialists had received their training there. Almost 50 percent of the practicing medical doctors in Texas had graduated from UTMB—4,500 of whom were still living. All had attended classes in Old Red. These facts and others helped ignite a movement to save the structure.[15]

With the future of Old Red in the balance, supporters of restoration proceeded in earnest. Led by Dr. E. Burke Evans, chief of orthopedic surgery at UTMB and president of the Galveston Historical Foundation, local supporters of preservation persuaded the regents to adopt a resolution to prevent the destruction of Old Red and to raise money for its restoration. However, the task of restoring Old Red promised to be a formidable one. While a feasibility study conducted by Wyatt C. Hedrick Architects and Engineers Inc. of Houston proclaimed Old Red to be structurally sound, portions of the building had degenerated. Investigators found sagging floors, warped wooden window frames, extreme cracks along the interior and exterior walls, severe deterioration in the mortar joints, and interior water damage. The initial price tag to restore the building was $2 million.[16]

The hefty amount needed to restore Old Red spurred considerable debate. It would cost far less, critics of preservation pointed out, to demolish the building than to save and renovate it. Besides, they asked, what usefulness did the old relic have within the modern campus environment? In the fall of 1972, Burke Evans issued a passionate rebuttal to such arguments in the *University Medical*:

> Persons who oppose preservation or who take no interest in it, tend to restrict their views to the present. Everything is judged in terms of current taste and current needs. The ugly Old Red Building should be torn down to make way for something modern we can use. The truth is, of course, that historic preservation is not for those who live but for those who are yet to live . . . The loss of a great building is like a death. Once it is gone, there is no way to replace

it. A picture will not do. Time dulls the pain and dims the memory. Succeeding generations will not miss it and life will go on perfectly well without it. This is either a chilling or a comforting fact. I am still sensitive to the possibility that the Red Building might not yet be saved and that others as foolish and romantic as I might not have the pleasure of its company.[17]

Two months after Evans published his appeal, UTMB President, Truman G. Blocker launched a vigorous fundraising campaign to restore Old Red that spanned the next ten years. In the process, preservation advocates ardently appealed to the UTMB community to get behind the "Save Old Red" cause. Early in the campaign, UTMB Dean Emeritus Chauncey D. Leake issued a particularly spirited plea to the alumni:

President Blocker's vision for saving this building need not be merely a pleasant dream: it can be, with vigorous and enthusiastic alumni support, a glorious reality ... Come on Alumni! Get behind President Blocker—or in front—with push, pull, and money! Get Old Red back in the game with us again, and the great ghost of its past will cheer![18]

And they did. Under Blocker's leadership and that of his successor, William C. Levin, UTMB alumni, faculty, and students supported the preservation campaign in numerous ways. They staged plays and sold red brick paperweights inscribed with a memorial picture of Old Red to secure funds. UTMB also produced an attractive brochure entitled "Old Red, Old Red" that described in poetry, photographs, and prose the vital role the building played throughout the history of the medical school. Texas citizens, the regular and the famous, also enrolled in the effort. Private supporters and benefactors included United States Senator and golf legend A. R. "Babe" Swartz, Houston civic leader Truett Latimer, Galveston County Judge Ray Holbrook, Galveston philanthropist Mary Moody Northen, and Peter Brink, executive director of the Galveston Historical Foundation. Latimer, who ranked Old Red in the same historical class as the Texas Capitol, the Governor's Mansion, and the Alamo, urged the regents to preserve and protect Old Red as a state treasure. In 1976 the Galveston County Bicentennial Committee recognized the preservation of Old Red as a state and national bicentennial project.[19]

Adding further momentum to the project, Chester R. Burns, Rockwell Professor of the History of Medicine at UTMB, published a paper answering on a historically factual basis, the question of why precisely

Old Red should be saved. After conducting a survey of medical schools throughout the United States, Burns discovered the following:

> Old Red is the oldest extant medical school building west of the Mississippi River and one of three extant nineteenth century buildings in the United States that once housed an entire medical school.
>
> It is the only extant nineteenth century medical school building west of the Mississippi River.
>
> It is the only medical school building of its kind that is designated as a historical landmark on the National Register of Historic Places and by the Texas Historical Commission.
>
> It is the only medical school building of its kind that embodies some of the special architectural styles of the late nineteenth century.

To summarize, Burns wrote, "The Ashbel Smith Building, of and by itself, is highly significant in American history and deserves preservation as a unique structure." It could therefore be affirmed that Old Red was a landmark memorial to medical education in Texas and to the nation.[20]

Despite enthusiastic appeals and fundraising efforts, the debate continued to swirl regarding whether salvaging Clayton's architectural jewel was worth the money to restore it. General inflation had sent construction costs skyward, while failing revenues had strained legislative allotments. By the late 1970s the estimate for total restoration of a building that originally cost $125,000 to build and equip in 1891, had risen to over $6 million. By July 1976, only $1 million had been committed for the restoration. Thus far, Presidents Blocker and Levin had been unsuccessful in convincing the regents to get behind Old Red. UTMB requested financial support for the restoration of Old Red from the Texas Legislature, but the request went unheeded. "No one wants to take it on," lamented Judge Ray Holbrook, "the restoration will take so much money . . . When I phoned legislators who were supposed to sponsor this bit of legislation to express my interest, they didn't even return my calls." Was it worth millions of dollars, the *Galveston Daily News* asked, to pull together a deteriorating fine old building ill-equipped to aid the work of modern science?[21]

In the end, two important factors saved Old Red. The first involved the acceptance of the "adaptive restoration" concept. In other words, Old Red could be preserved, yet modified to meet the contemporary requirements of UTMB. That caveat coupled with the Medical Branch tradition of blending state resources with private philanthropy won the day. Architects carefully planned the restored space with a clear view of the history and legacies associated with the building. The department of anatomy was given laboratory and classroom space at its original site. The gross anatomy laboratory, with its multitude of specimens that had intrigued freshmen medical students for almost a century, was also restored. Two newcomers to the building were the Graduate School of Biological Sciences and the Institute for the Medical Humanities. In 1973 the Medical Branch became one of very few medical schools in the United States to create a program committed to the study and teaching of the humanities from a medical perspective. A variety of courses addressing medical history, philosophy, religion, and ethics were incorporated into the medical curriculum at UTMB. To many at UTMB, Old Red was the perfect setting for students to explore medicine's past while addressing the human medical needs of the future.[22]

A turning point for the restoration campaign occurred in October 1978, when the University of Texas Board of Regents voted to restore Old Red. A key factor in the regent endorsement involved a surprise telegram to the regents from Galveston philanthropist Mary Moody Northen. In the announcement, Northen offered on behalf of the Moody Foundation a $500,000 challenge grant in support of the preservation effort. Calling the restoration of Old Red "a necessity," the board matched the offer with $1 million from the Permanent University Fund. The Moody Foundation pledge, combined with other private donations, added $1.6 million to the project. Then, in September 1980, after UTMB President Levin made an impassioned appeal for additional support, the regents allocated another $5 million for the restoration of Old Red. The amount offered was based upon the projected equivalent of new construction of the same space.

Two years later, the regents approved plans for a three-phase refurbishment of Old Red. The first phase of the process involved stabilizing and restoring of the building exterior. The installation of elevators, fire stairs, updated plumbing, and electrical work took place in the second phase. The final portion of the project addressed the beautiful interior. Architects maintained the historical integrity of the building by restoring the high ceilings and detail in the amphitheater, large classrooms, and corridors, while installing modern office space in other areas of the building. In the summer of 1985, contractors added the final touches to Old Red, and new tenants began to move in. The student affairs office and a student lounge occupied the first floor. The second floor was reserved for the Graduate School of Biomedical Sciences and the Institute for the Medical Humanities, along with the beautifully restored amphitheater. The third floor, inclusive of a skylit dissection lab, became the territory of the Department of Anatomy.[23]

Formal rededication ceremonies for Old Red were held on April 10,

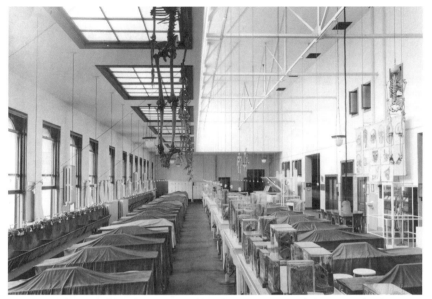

Restored anatomy lab with specimens, Old Red (1990s). *Courtesy Blocker History of Medicine Collections, Moody Medical Library.*

1986. Regent Jane Weinert Blumberg proclaimed the beautifully restored structure a symbol that "renews ties with the past while giving us the strength to go forward." As employees and students ascended the magnificent Texas pine and mahogany staircase, meandered through the long, spacious hallways, and took their seats in classrooms and offices, Clayton's masterpiece once again became a fully functioning part of UTMB. First-year medical students performed anatomy dissections surrounded by more than five hundred jars of human specimens that lined the shelves of the high-ceilinged room. On the floor directly below, individuals seeking degrees in the medical humanities attended lectures in the steeply sloped amphitheater or smaller classrooms warmed by large, beautifully arched windows. However, the legacy of Old Red was perhaps best symbolized on the first floor. Upon entering the large, blue front doors, UTMB faculty, students, and visitors were immediately flanked by a series of impressive statues by sculptor Doris Appel. A gift of Houston physician and philanthropist John P. McGovern, the McGovern Hall of Medical History displayed the plaster-cast images of eleven medical pioneers, from Imhotep to Marie Curie, who epitomized centuries of caregiving, teaching, and the everlasting quest for scientific knowledge.[24]

Since the restoration, those who have studied and worked inside Old

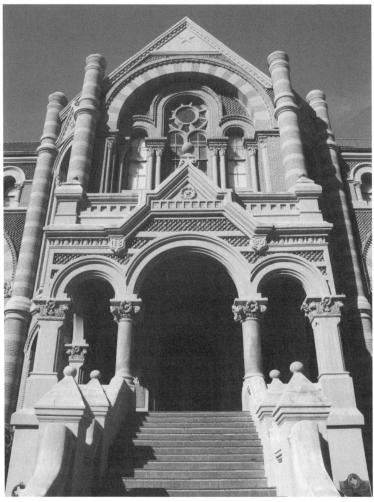

Old Red restored front view (2011). *Courtesy Lisa Reyna.*

Red have felt a profound presence unobtainable anywhere else at UTMB. "Stepping into Old Red was like stepping into history," remembered UTMB alumnus Lynnette A. Masters (class of 2006), "knowing that so many have walked the path before you." Students attending lectures or laboring in the dissection lab were proud in the belief that they were carrying on a great century-old tradition. However, for many, Old Red has also provided a measure of peace in the midst of the high-stress medical school environment. "There was comfort in knowing Old Red had survived so much," asserted Masters, "The people who walked the halls had survived so much, and so could I."[25] The time spent for students inside Old Red was brief—a mere transition period before moving on to a profession in medicine. Whenever they are in Galveston, UTMB alumni often make their way back to Old Red. Many are now gray-headed and move a bit slower. But they find solace and pleasure both in their treasured memories of Old Red and the promises it holds for future generations.

EPILOGUE

FOR MORE THAN TWENTY YEARS after its restoration, the Ashbel Smith Building remained untouched by natural or manmade disaster. But a huge setback occurred on September 13, 2008, when Hurricane Ike blanketed the Island with floodwaters causing millions of dollars' worth of damage to UTMB campus buildings, hospitals, and clinics. More than eight feet of water poured into the ground floor of Old Red, destroying the morgue on one end, a beautiful new faculty lounge on the other, and offices for the UTMB Willed Body Program and Student Affairs in the middle. The damage compelled an immediate closing of the landmark. Gross Anatomy, the Institute for the Medical Humanities, Student Enrollment Services, and other offices moved elsewhere on campus.

The absence of life inside Old Red was only temporary. In the months following the storm, UTMB ordered a condition assessment of Old Red, whereby the building was proclaimed structurally sound. As of 2012, the first two floors of Old Red have been completely reoccupied by Enrollment Services and Student Affairs offices. Lectures and other events have resumed in the east amphitheater.

Subsequent phases will determine use of the ground and third floors. After ground floor building systems and equipment have been permanently moved out of harm's way, the ground floor space is expected to be used for informal student services, including study areas, a student lounge, and other venues. Plans for the third floor involve the creation of a medical history museum, highlighting some of Old Red's most famous possessions—the rows of pathology specimen jars—as its focal point.

OLD RED TIMELINE

1881 Seventeenth Texas Legislature voted to establish the University of Texas and Medical Department.

1888 Nicholas J. Clayton commissioned to design the structure that would house the new medical school.

1891 October 5: Medical Department opened for its first academic session.

1892 April 22: The first three graduates received diplomas from the Medical Department.

1900 September 8: Storm of the century caused severe damage to Old Red. Two months later, classes resumed.

1909 Abraham Flexner visited Medical Department and gave it a high ranking in the 1910 Flexner Report.

1915 Hurricane swept across Galveston but the newly constructed seawall and grade-raising project prevent the disastrous circumstances of 1900.

1916 December 9: Nicholas Clayton died.

1919 University of Texas Medical Department renamed UT Medical Branch.

1942 UTMB placed on probation.

1943 September: Probation period lifted.

1949   Old Red dedicated as the Ashbel Smith Building.

1961   Hurricane Carla caused extensive damage to Old Red.

1966   Old Red scheduled for demolition.

1986   April 10: Old Red officially rededicated after four-year restoration.

2008   September 13: Hurricane Ike flooded Old Red causing damage. Old Red closed.

2011   Old Red reopened.

Notes

Chapter 1

[1] Elizabeth Silverthorne, *Ashbel Smith of Texas* (College Station: Texas A&M University Press, 1982), 218.

[2] Chester R. Burns, "Health and Medicine," The Handbook of Texas Online, <http://www.tshaonline.org/handbook/online/articles/HH/smhzc.html> [Accessed May 27, 2010]; James H. Cassedy, *Medicine in America: A Short History* (Baltimore: Johns Hopkins University Press, 1991), 89; Ralph Edwards, "Health and Medical Care at the Time of the American Centennial," *Journal of School Health* 66 (February 1976): 77–78.

[3] Burns, "Health and Medicine," *The Handbook of Texas Online.*

[4] Cassedy, *Medicine in America*, 29, 42; David McCullough, *The Greater Journey: Americans in Paris* (New York; Simon & Schuster, 2011), 105–106; Silverthorne, *Ashbel Smith of Texas*, 23–24.

[5] Kenneth Ludmerer, *Learning to Heal: The Development of American Medical Education* (Baltimore: Johns Hopkins University Press, 1996), 38.

[6] Edwards, "Health and Medical Care at the Time of the American Centennial," 78–79.

[7] Susan Reverby, *Ordered to Care: The Dilemma of American Nursing, 1850–1900* (Cambridge, UK: Cambridge University Press, 1987), 22.

[8] Heather Green Campbell, "A Note on the First Nursing School in Texas and its Role in the Nineteenth Century American Experience," *The Houston Review* 19, No. 1 (1997): 51.

[9] Larry Wygant, "Medicine and Public Health in Galveston, Texas: The First Century" (Ph.D. diss., University of Texas Medical Branch, 1992), 203–204.

[10] *Galveston News,* July 3, 1855.

[11] Larry Wygant, "A Sickly City: Health and Disease in Antebellum Galveston, Texas," *Houston Review* 19, No. 1 (1997) 27.

[12] Wygant, "A Sickly City," 29.

[13] Wygant, "A Sickly City," 28.

[14] Andrew Forest Muir (ed.), *Texas in 1837: An Anonymous Contemporary Narrative* (Austin: University of Texas Press, 1958), 132.

[15] Heather Green Campbell, "The Yellow Pestilence: A Comparative Study of the 1853 Yellow Fever Epidemic in New Orleans and the Galveston, Texas Scourge of 1867," *East Texas Historical Journal* 37 (January 1999): 5.

[16] Wygant, "Medicine and Public Health in Galveston," 28–30.

[17] Ashbel Smith, *Yellow Fever in Galveston, Republic of Texas, 1839* (reprint, Austin: University of Texas Press, 1951), 42; Campbell, "The Yellow Pestilence," 5–6; Wygant, "A Sickly City," 29–31; Silverthorne, *Ashbel Smith of Texas,* 60–62.

[18] Lucy P. Shaw to Jane N. Weston, Dec. 3, 1839, Lucy P. Shaw Papers, MS 24-0043

(Galveston and Texas History Center, Rosenberg Library, Galveston, Texas; cited hereafter as GTHC).

[19] Wygant, "A Sickly City," 32–34.

[20] Charles Hooten, *St. Louis Isle, or Texiana: With Additional Observations Made in the United States and in Canada* (London: Simmonds & Ward, 1847), 38.

[21] Wygant, "Medicine and Public Health in Galveston, Texas," 145.

[22] Sister Mary Loyola Hegarty, *Serving with Gladness: The Origin and History of the Congregation of the Sisters of Charity of the Incarnate Word* (Houston: Bruce Publishing Co., 1967), 200.

[23] Elizabeth Silverthorne and Geneva Fulgham, *Women Pioneers in Texas Medicine* (College Station: Texas A&M University Press, 1997), 48–51.

[24] Ralph W. Jones, "The First Roots of the University of Texas Medical Branch at Galveston," *Southwestern Historical Quarterly* 65 (April 1962): 465–66; *The University of Texas Medical Branch at Galveston: A Seventy-Five Year History by the Faculty and Staff* (Austin: University of Texas Press, 1967; cited hereafter as *Seventy-Five Year History*), 5–6. Many antebellum physicians in the South were advocates of "states' rights," not only in terms of slavery, but also medical therapeutics. Southern physicians contended that geographic differences made the South so distinctive that medical practice, as taught in northern medical schools, was virtually useless in the treatment of "Southern diseases." John Harley Warner, "The Idea of Southern Medical Distinctiveness: Medical Knowledge and Practice in the Old South," in Judith Walzer Leavitt and Ronald L. Numbers (eds.), *Sickness and Health in America* (2nd ed.; Madison: University of Wisconsin Press, 1985), 53–70.

[25] Gary Cartwright, *Galveston: A History of the Island* (Fort Worth: TCU Press, 1991), 119–120; T. R. Fehrenbach, *Lone Star: A History of Texas and Texans* (New York: Collier Books, 1986), 601; Tom Hunter, *The House of Honored Men, A Story of Three Prominent Galvestonians, The City They Called Home, and The Bishop's Palace* (Galveston: The Bishop's Palace, 1998), 55–57.

[26] The Galveston City Directory for 1875–1876 lists fifty-two physicians.

[27] Chester R. Burns, *Saving Lives, Training Caregivers, Making Discoveries: A Centennial History of the University of Texas Medical Branch at Galveston* (Austin: Texas State Historical Association, 2003), 10–11.

[28] Inci Bowman, "Beginnings of Medical Journalism in Texas," *Texas Medicine* 82 (February 1986): 51.

[29] *Seventy-Five Year History*, 7.

[30] James Fannin Young (J. F. Y.) Paine, "Opening Address to the Medical Department," *University Medical* 11 (October 1906): 3–6.

[31] *Seventy-Five Year History*, 8.

[32] Jones, "First Roots of the Medical Branch," 470.

[33] Burns, *Saving Lives*, 11–12.

[34] *Special Laws of the State of Texas* (1871), Texas State Library and Archives, Austin, 499–501; Burns, *Saving Lives*, 11–13; *Seventy-five Year History*, 7–9.

[35] Richard Cole, "The Regent Who Bellowed Fire," *Alcalde* 53 (April 1965): 25.

[36] Silverthorne, *Ashbel Smith of Texas*, 218.

[37] David G. McComb, *Galveston: A History and Guide* (Austin: Texas State Historical Association, 2000), 17–18; David G. McComb, *Galveston: A History* (Austin: University of Texas Press, 1986), 98; Chester R. Burns, "The University of Texas Medical Branch at Galveston: Origins and Beginnings," *Journal of the American Medical Association* 266 (Sept. 11, 1991), 1401; Silverthorne, *Ashbel Smith of Texas*, 210–212.

[38] Burns, *Saving Lives*, 16–17; *Seventy-Five Year History*, 15.

[39] Pat Ireland Nixon, *A History of the Texas Medical Association, 1853–1953* (Austin: University of Texas Press, 1953), 97.

[40] Nixon, *A History of the Texas Medical Association*, 93–94.

[41] Campbell, "A Note on the First Nursing School in Texas," 49–51; Silverthorne and Fulgham, *Women Pioneers*, 34–35.

[42] Burns, *Saving Lives*, 20–21.

[43] Campbell, "A Note on the First Nursing School in Texas," 55; Silverthorne and Fulgham, *Women Pioneers*, 35.

Chapter 2

[1] Barrie Scardino and Drexel Turner, *Clayton's Galveston* (College Station: Texas A&M University Press, 2000), 29; 260n2; Pauline Jackson, Pauline Jackson, "Women in 19th Century Irish Immigration," *International Migration Review* 18 (Winter 1984): 1004–1005; Edward Oxford, "The Great Famine," *American History* 31 (March–April 1996): 52–58.

[2] Robert A. Nesbitt and Stephen Fox, "Nicholas Joseph Clayton," *The Handbook of Texas Online*, http://w.w.w.tshaonline.org/handbook/online/article/CC/fc122_print.html [Accessed Sept. 16, 2009]; Howard Barnstone, *The Galveston That Was* (Houston: Rice University Press, 1966), 79–81; Scardino and Turner, *Clayton's Galveston*, 29.

[3] Scardino and Turner, *Clayton's Galveston*, 30–31.

[4] Ibid. 30.

[5] Ibid. 31.

[6] Tom Hunter, *The House of Honored Men*, 21; Bob Parvin, "Nicholas Clayton: The Image-Maker of Texas' Victorian Pageant," *Texas Highways* 27 (January 1980): 17.

[7] Robert A. Nesbitt, "The Legend of Nicholas Clayton," *Port Galveston* 27, No. 6 (1974): 10–11; Parvin, "Nicholas Clayton," 18–19; Hunter, *The House of Honored Men,* 21; *Galveston Daily News*, Dec. 10, 1874.

[8] Nesbitt, "The Legend of Nicholas Clayton," 14–15; "Nicholas J. Clayton," *Galveston Daily News*, Feb. 20, 1972.

[9] "Nicholas J. Clayton," *Galveston Daily News,* Feb. 20, 1972; Cleta Sireno, "Mary Clayton: For more than 50 years she has recorded the histories of Galvestonians on film," *Galveston Daily News,* Apr. 22, 1982; Scardino and Turner, *Clayton's Galveston*, 125–126.

[10] Nesbitt and Fox, "Nicholas Joseph Clayton" *Handbook of Texas Online*; Scardino and Turner, *Clayton's Galveston*, 40, 80.

[11] Daybook, 1887, Nicholas J. Clayton Papers, 1874–1915, Box 1 (GTHC).

[12] Nesbitt, "The Legend of Nicholas Clayton," 14l; Scardino and Turner, *Clayton's Galveston*, 152–153.

[13] Robert Nesbitt, "Nicholas J. Clayton (1839–1916): Galveston's Great Architect," unpublished manuscript, 27, (Galveston Country Historical Commission Archives, Galveston, Texas).

[14] Daybook, Dec. 20, 1887 (GTHC).

[15] Nesbitt, "Nicholas Clayton," 24–25; Parvin, "Nicholas Clayton," 19–20; Scardino and Turner, *Clayton's Galveston,* 124–125.

[16] Hunter, *The House of Honored Men*, 39–53. Additional information regarding Galveston's pleasure palaces can be found in Scardino and Turner, *Clayton's Galveston*, 49–53, 83–85.

[17] Barnstone, *The Galveston That Was*, 79; Cartwright, *Galveston: A History of the Island,* 147.

[18] Ellen Beasley and Stephen Fox, *Galveston: Architecture Guidebook* (Houston: Rice University Press and the Galveston Historical Foundation, 1996), 47–48, 52–53, 110–111, 172, 175–176.

[19] "Mary Clayton," *Galveston Daily News*, Apr. 22, 1982; Parvin, "Nicholas Clayton," 20–21.

[20] Nesbitt, "The Legend of Nicholas Clayton," 10-11; Scardino and Turner, *Clayton's*

Galveston, 224. For an overview of Texas churches including Clayton contributions in Galveston, see Willard B. Robinson, "Houses of Worship in Nineteenth-Century Texas," *Southwestern Historical Quarterly* 85 (January 1982): 235–298.

[21] Willard B. Robinson, *Texas Public Buildings of the Nineteenth Century* (Austin: University of Texas Press, 1974), 144–146; Willard B. Robinson, "Temples of Knowledge: Historic Mains of Texas Colleges and Universities," *Southwestern Historical Quarterly* 77 (April 1974): 462.

[22] "Special Council Meeting to Secure Medical Branch," *Galveston Daily News*, Feb. 15, 1887; Apr. 16, 1888; Sept. 3, 1888; Sept. 17, 1889, Regents Minutes, UT Board of Regents Offices, Ashbel Smith Hall, University of Texas at Austin; Burns, *Saving Lives,* 17–18.

[23] Regents Minutes, Sept. 17, 1889. First quotation from J. J. Lane, *History of the University of Texas* (Austin: Hutchings, 1891), 168; Second quotation from Nicholas J. Clayton to UT Regents, Dec. 9, 1890, letter reprinted as "Exhibit O," *Alcalde* 4 (December 1890): 54.

[24] Drexel Turner, "Construction and Architecture of the Ashbel Smith Building," *The Bookman*, 6 (March, 1979), 4–5; "Contract Awarded," *Galveston Daily News*, Oct. 13, 1889; Burns, *Saving Lives*, 18–19.

[25] "The Medical Branch," *Galveston Daily News*, June 23, 1889; Turner, "Construction and Architecture of the Ashbel Smith Building," 6–7; Scardino and Turner, *Clayton's Galveston*, 95–99; Lawrence W. Speck and Richard Payne, *Landmarks of Texas Architecture* (Austin: University of Texas Press, 1986), 40–43.

[26] Scardino and Turner, *Clayton's Galveston*, 127–134.

[27] Quotation from Barnstone, *The Galveston That Was*, 161. The gravesite of Nicholas Clayton now contains two markers. One is a small headstone. The other is a tall monument bearing his name.

Chapter 3

[1] *Seventy-Five Year History*, 51; Burns, *Saving Lives*, 21.

[2] Allen J. Smith, "Beginning of the Medical Department Memories," *Alcalde* 3 (July 1915): 742.

[3] Seth Mabry Morris, "Opening Address," *University Medical* 41 (December 1936): 4.

[4] Smith, "Beginning of the Medical Department Memories," 742.

[5] *Seventy-Five Year History*, 27.

[6] Ibid.

[7] James E. Thompson, "The University Stops for No Storm," *Galveston Tribune*, June 5, 1925. For a detailed description of the outstanding careers of William Keiller and James Edwin Thompson, see Chester R. Burns and Heather Green Campbell, "Two Extraordinary Influences of Two British Physicians on Medical Education and Practice in Texas at the Turn of the 20th Century," *Vesalius* 5 (December 1999): 79–84.

[8] Smith, "Beginning of the Medical Department Memories," 745.

[9] *Report of the UT Board of* Regents (1890), 3–4; (1892), 5–6, cited in Burns, *Saving Lives*, 19.

[10] Thompson, "The University Stops for No Storm."

[11] H. L. Hilgartner, "Life, Character and Works of Professor J. W. McLaughlin," *Texas Medical Journal* 15 (June 1910): 562.

[12] Morris, "Opening Address," 10.

[13] Thompson, "The University Stops for No Storm."

[14] William Keiller, "Opening Address of the Medical Department, October 3, 1893," *University Medical* 3 (January 1898): 97.

[15] Burns, *Saving Lives*, 37.

[16] *Seventy-Five Year History*, 45.

[17] Campbell, "A Note on the First Nursing School in Texas," 55; *Seventy-Five Year History*, 68–69.

[18] Burns, *Saving Lives*, 27; *Seventy-Five Year History*, 68–69.

[19] Wygant, "Medicine and Public Health in Galveston," 77.

[20] Morris, "Opening Address," 4.

[21] West authored twenty-seven medical papers on the study of typhoid, dysentery, dengue, and yellow fevers, and he was cited for his observations in William Osler's premier work, *The Principles and Practice of Medicine* (1892).

[22] H. R. Dudgeon, "Random Undergraduate Recollections," *Alcalde* 3 (July 1915): 853–855; *Seventy-Five Year History*, 32.

[23] R. L. Wilson, "Recollections of School Days, 1895–1899, Medical Department University of Texas," *Alcalde* 3 (July 1915): 854.

[24] Megan Seaholm, "The Students and Student Life at the University of Texas Medical Department in Galveston, 1891–1901" (unpublished manuscript), 9–10, Centennial History Project (hereafter cited as CHP), Series 13, Box 39, File: Student Life (Blocker History of Medicine Collections, Moody Medical Library, Galveston, Texas; cited hereafter as BHMC); J. R. Elliott, "History [of class of '01]," *Cactus* 5 (1898): 72–73; Dudgeon, "Random Undergraduate Recollections," 857–858.

[25] William Keiller, "William Spencer Carter," *Alcalde* 10 (June 1922): 1403.

[26] Morris, "Opening Address," 4.

[27] "The Representation of the Medical Department in the Spanish-American War," *University Record* 1 (April 1899): 139; Wilson, "Recollections of School Days," 854.

[28] Thompson, "The University Stops for No Storm."

[29] *Seventy-Five Year History*, 54. Now demolished, Harmony Hall was located at Twenty-First and Church Streets.

[30] Burns, *Saving Lives*, Appendix P, 439.

[31] "The Opening of the Medical Department," *University Record* 2 (December 1900): 383–385.

[32] Allen J. Smith, "The Medical Department and the Galveston Storm," *University Record* 3 (March 1901): 56.

[33] Quotes from Dudgeon, "Random Undergraduate Recollections," 859–860. For a concise account of the 1900 storm, see David G. McComb, *Galveston: A History* (Austin: University of Texas Press, 1986), 121–133.

[34] "Nicholas J. Clayton", *Galveston Daily News*, Feb. 20, 1972.

[35] "The Great Storm at Galveston—From a Medical Standpoint" *Texas Medical Journal* 16 (1901): 166.

[36] C. T. Peckham, Surgeon, U.S.M.H.S. "Report of the Tornado at Galveston, September 11, 1900," *Public Health Reports* 15 (1900): 2376.

[37] Smith, "The Medical Department and the Galveston Storm," 57(first quotation); 60 (second and third quotations); 63 (fourth quotation).

[38] Patricia Bellis Bixel and Elizabeth Hayes Turner, *Galveston and the 1900 Storm* (Austin: University of Texas Press, 2000), 70–71; McComb, *Galveston: A History*, 135.

[39] Jodi Wright-Gidley and Jennifer Marines, *Galveston: A City on Stilts* (Charleston S.C.: Arcadia Publishing, 2008), 11; Bixel and Turner, *Galveston and the 1900 Storm*, 106; McComb, *Galveston: A History*, 141–143.

[40] W. S. Carter to W. L. Prather, Jan. 28, 1905, CHP, Series 4, Box 13, File: Community Faculty Life (BHMC).

[41] Advertisement, *Texas State Journal of Medicine* 5 (May 1909): 12. The ad was published to herald an upcoming Texas State Medical Association meeting in Galveston. It most likely bore an influence since over eight hundred individuals attended. See Burns, *Savings Lives*, 358.

[42] Thompson, "The University of Texas Stops for No Storm," *Galveston Tribune*, June 5, 1925; *Seventy-Five Year History*, 122–123.

[43] Minutes, University of Texas Board of Regents, Sept. 17, 1900, CHP, Box 27, File: Unpublished Minutes UTMB Board of Regents: 1900–1906 (BHMC); *Seventy-Five Year History*, 62.

[44] Thompson, "The University of Texas Stops for No Storm." When the school's first trained librarian, Kate Feuille, arrived at UTMB in 1920, the medical school library boasted over ten thousand volumes. *Seventy-Five Year History*, 122–123.

[45] Allen J. Smith, "The First Decade," Opening Address to the Medical Department, *University Medical* 6 (October 1901): 8.

[46] "A Negro Hospital: One of the Finest in the South," *Galveston Daily News*, Apr. 6, 1902.

[47] Heather Green Wooten, *The Polio Years in Texas: Battling a Terrifying Unknown* (College Station: Texas A&M University Press, 2009), 190–91n 45.

[48] Burns, *Saving Lives*, 359; William S. Carter, "A Decade of Progress in the Medical Department in its Beginning," *Alcalde* 3 (July 1915): 745.

[49] Abraham Flexner, *Medical Education in the United States and Canada: A Report to the Carnegie Foundation for the Advancement of Teaching* (Boston: The Merrymount Press, 1910), 312.

[50] Ibid.

[51] Ibid., 311.

[52] Ibid, 312.

[53] W. S. Carter, "A Decade of Progress in the Medical Department," *Alcalde* 2 (March 1914): 459. For an excellent history of medical education in the United States, including the nation-wide ramifications of the Flexner Report, see Kenneth M. Ludmerer, *Learning to Heal: The Development of American Medical Education* (Baltimore: Johns Hopkins University Press, 1985

[54] *Seventy-Five Year History*, 112.

[55] Flexner, *Medical Education in the United States and Canada*, 312.

[56] Burns, *Saving Lives*, 42–43.

[57] Thomas H. Nolan to W. J. Battle, telegram, Aug. 19, 1915 cited in *Seventy-Five Year History*, 108–109.

[58] C. B. Carter, "Forty Years of Surgery in the University of Texas Medical Branch, 1915–1955," (transcript), quoted in *Seventy-Five Year History*, 107.

[59] T. T. Jackson, "Going Back to Galveston," *Alcalde* 4 (June 1916): 766–767.

[60] Bryan Boutwell and John P. McGovern, *Conversation with a Medical School: The University of Texas-Houston Medical School, 1970–2000* (Houston: University of Texas at Houston, 1999), 71.

[61] Burns, *Saving Lives*, 42–43.

[62] Ralph Steen, "World War I," *The Handbook of Texas Online*, http://www.tshaonline. org/handbook/online/articles/qdw01 [Accessed Apr. 6, 2012]; Quotation: *Houston Post*, July 9, 1917, cited in Patrick L. Cox, "An Enemy Closer to Us than Any European Power": The Impact of Mexico on Texan Public Opinion before World War I," *Southwestern Historical Quarterly* 105 (July 2001): 78–79.

[63] "Medical Men as Volunteers," *South Texas Medical Record* 11 (July 1917): 7.

[64] Harry O. Knight, "Opening Address to the Medical Department," *University Medical* 22 (November 1917): 8.

[65] *Seventy-Five Year History*, 109; Julia Williams Bertner Naylor Interview to Don Macon, July 19, 1973 (interview), Ernst W. Bertner, M.D., Papers, Series 2, Box 1, Folder 3; William D. Seybold, "E. W. Bertner, M.D., F.A.C.S." (unpublished manuscript), 3–4, Bertner Papers, Series 2, Box 1, Folder 7, John P. McGovern History of Medicine Collections, Houston Research Center-Texas Medical Center.

[66] *Seventy-Five Year History*, 109; quotes from Howard O. Smith, "The Years 1918–1922" (transcript), 2–3, Seventy-Five Year History Files, MS 15, Box 1, File: Alumni Reminiscences (BHMC).

[67] Burns, *Savings Lives*, 44.

[68] W. H. Dougherty to R. E. Vinson, May 20, 1920, CHP, Series 7, Box 27, File: Records of the President–UT Austin (BHMC).

[69] "News," *Texas State Journal of Medicine* 16 (July 1920): 138; "Medical College Committee Named," *Galveston Daily News*, Sept. 9, 1920.

[70] "Excellent Site for the Medical School Is Found at Galveston, Maintain Witnesses," *Galveston Daily News*, Nov. 5, 1920.

[71] Attorney General to Honorable Leonard Tillotson in Sealy, Texas, Nov. 22, 1920, Sealy and Smith Foundation, Board of Directors, "Historical Review of the Medical Branch of the University of Texas and of the Sealy and Smith Foundation for the John Sealy Hospital at Galveston," 21 (BHMC); "Report on the Medical College," *Galveston Daily News*, Dec. 28, 1920.

[72] David G. McComb, "Galveston: A Tourist City," *Southwestern Historical Quarterly* 100 (January 1997): 344–345; McComb, *Galveston: A History*, 180–181.

[73] Advertisement, *Texas State Journal of Medicine* 23 (April 1928): 808–809.

[74] Burns, *Saving Lives*, 76; Sealy & Smith Foundation for the John Sealy Hospital, Report 1922–1972, CHP, Series 8, Box 30, File: Sealy and Smith Foundation; "Committee Favors Holbrook Measure: Would Give Sealy Inheritance Tax To Galveston Hospital," *Galveston Daily News*, Sept. 24, 1926; "Real Estate Transfers," *Galveston Daily News*, Oct. 5, 1926.

[75] Burns, *Saving Lives*, 76.

[76] Burns, *Saving Lives*, 108–109.

[77] "New Hospital for Crippled Children to be Built Here: Federal Funds Sought for New Hospital for Negroes," *Galveston Daily News*, Jan. 16, 1936; "Hospital for Crippled Children to be Erected Here," *Galveston Daily News*, Jan. 19, 1936; *Seventy-Five Year History*, 149–150.

[78] Burns, *Saving Lives*, 364; *Seventy-Five Year History*, 157.

[79] *Seventy-Five Year History*, 163.

[80] Frederick C. Elliott, William H. Kellar, and Richard E. Wainerdi, *The Birth of the Texas Medical Center: A Personal Account* (College Station: Texas A&M University Press, 2004), 9.

[81] Ibid., 10–11.

[82] Meagan Seaholm, "Student Life at the University of Texas Medical Branch, 1942–1966," unpublished manuscript, 2, CHP, Series 13, Box 39, File: Seaholm: UTMB Student Life: 1942–1966 (BHMC).

[83] Burns, *Saving Lives*, 52–53; Elliott, Kellar, and Wainerdi, *The Birth of the Texas Medical Center*, 11.

[84] Denton A. Cooley to Chester R. Burns, Sept., 4, 1987, cited in Seaholm, "Student Life at the University of Texas Medical Branch, 1942–1966," 2.

[85] Minutes, UT Board of Regents, Feb. 28, 1942, cited in Burns, *Saving Lives*, 52–53.

[86] *Seventy-Five Year History*, 168.

[87] Denton A. Cooley, review of *Saving Lives, Training Caregivers, Making Discoveries: A Centennial History of the University of Texas Medical Branch at Galveston*, by Chester R. Burns, *Texas Heart Institute Journal* 30, no. 4 (2003): 342–343.

[88] Chauncey D. Leake to J. C. Geiger, Sept. 19, 1942 (first quotation); Chauncey D. Leake to Robert Gordon Sproul, Oct. 20, 1942 (second quotation) both cited in Burns, *Savings Lives*, 54–55; *Seventy-Five Year History*, 170.

[89] Thomas O. Shindler, "Personal Impressions, The University of Texas Medical Branch, The War Years and Afterwards, 1940–1950" (transcript), MS 15, Box 1, File: Alumni Reminiscences (BHMC).

[90] *Seventy-Five Year History*, 291–293.

[91] Schindler, "Personal Impressions, the University of Texas Medical Branch," 2–3.

[92] *Seventy-Five Year History*, 174–177.

[93] Seaholm, "Student Life the University of Texas Medical Branch, 1942–1966," 12–13.

[94] "Graduating Exercises for 143 Medical and Nursing Students Set for Tomorrow," Unidentified news clipping, June 23, 2943; UTMB Scrapbook, 1942–1949; "Medical Students Receive Orders from Navy" (news clipping), June 30, 1943; "Army Gives Military Training to 150 Students at Medical School," unidentified news clipping, July 25, 1943; UTMB Scrapbook, 1942–1949 (BHMC).

[95] *Seventy-Five Year History*, 177.

[96] "Plans for Army Medical Hospital Confirmed," *Galveston Daily News*, Feb. 3, 1942. Further details of the 127th campaign can be found in Robert Moore (ed.), "The 127th General Hospital" (unpublished manuscript), 1949, Rare Book Room (BHMC); the World War II Alumni Collection of newspaper clippings and Overseas Letters, Mildred Robertson Papers (BHMC); Burns, *Saving Lives*, 320–321.

[97] *The 127th General Hospital: Activated 1943; Inactivated 1945* (np: nd), 13.

[98] "Polio Patients in Galveston Felt Near Misses in Storm," *Dallas Morning News*, Aug. 1, 1946; Ted Streuli, "The Mystery Storm of 1943," *Galveston Daily News*, July 27, 2003.

[99] Mason Freeman, "Gulf Coast Hurricane Hits U.T. Med School," *Daily Texan*, Aug. 1, 1943; Chauncey D. Leake to Homer P. Rainey, Memo, July 29, 1943, CHP, Series 4, Box 13, File: Hurricanes and Their Impact (BHMC); *Seventy-Five Year History*, 209–210.

[100] Chauncey D. Leake to T. S. Painter, Aug. 28, 1945, School of Nursing Archives, Dean's Correspondence, Box 1, File 6 (BHMC).

[101] In Vinsant's hometown of San Benito, Texas, a hospital, the Dolly Vinsant Memorial Hospital, was named in her memory. In a postwar ceremony, President Harry Truman posthumously awarded Vinsant a purple heart and a personal citation for bravery. Silverthorne, *Women Pioneers in Texas Medicine*, 46–48.

[102] Cassedy, *Medicine in America*, 126.

[103] Allie Fay Mosbee, "Students Give Disaster Service in Galveston," *American Journal of Nursing* 47 (June 1947): 414.

[104] Seaholm, "Student Life the University of Texas Medical Branch, 1942–1966," 5–6.

[105] Silverthorne, *Women Pioneers*, 172.

[106] *Seventy-Five Year History*, 180.

[107] Burns, *Saving Lives*, 148; Maureen Bayless Balleza, "Center of Excellence," *Galveston Daily News*, Aug. 21, 2012.

[108] A native of Brooklyn, New York, Panderewski had resided in Galveston two years when he received the commission to create the Smith bust. He was a trained artist and musician: During those years he was a sculptor by day and played cello evenings with the Houston Symphony. Panderewski eventually devoted many years of his career to constructing prosthetic parts for human faces at the Shriners Burns Institute at UTMB. "Memorial to be Erected: 92 Doctors, Nurses to Get Degrees at Pier Exercises," *Galveston Daily News*, June 5, 1949; "Bust of Dr. Ashbel Smith Unveiled at Medical Branch," *Galveston Daily News*, June 11, 1949; Hal Wimberly, "Sculptor's Art Aid to Hospital," *Houston Chronicle*, Aug. 14, 1960.

Chapter 4

[1] Less than one quarter of the student population came from counties that included large cities: Galveston, Bexar, Harris, Dallas, and Travis. Megan Seaholm, "Student Life at the University of Texas Medical Branch, 1901–1941" (unpublished manuscript), 8–10, CHP, Series 13, Box 39, File: Student Life, 1891–1941 (BHMC).

[2] Meagan Seaholm, "Student Life at the University of Texas Medical Department, 1891–1901," 6–7, CHP, Series 13, Box 39, File: Seaholm, Student Life at the University of Texas

Medical Department, 1891–1941 (BHMC). In 1897 the School of Nursing catalogue stated "It is the intention of the authorities to eventually admit both sexes when the size of the hospital will permit." However, it was not until the 1950s that the first male students were admitted to the school, and none graduated until 1963. *Seventy-Five Year History*, 94–95.

³ Seaholm, Student Life at the University of Texas Medical Department, 1901–1941," 10–13; Burns, *Saving Lives*, 27; Silverthorne and Fulgham, *Women Pioneers*, 36.

⁴ "Quartet of Physicians Had Served College 35 Years," *Galveston Daily News*, Apr. 4, 1926 (quotation); "Pioneering Spirit Marked Original Medical Faculty," *Galveston Daily News,* Apr. 4, 1926; *Seventy-Five Year History*, 54, 64.

⁵ *Seventy-Five Year History*, 93.

⁶ Megan Seaholm, "Student Life at the University of Texas Medical Department, 1901–1941," 2–3. Catalogues of the Department of Medicine of the University of Texas, Galveston, Texas: 1891–92, 6–7; 1892–93, 7–8; 1893–94, 6–7; 1894–95, 11–14; 1895–96, 12–16; 1896–97, 13–16; 1897–98, 16–20; 1898–99, 15–19; 1899–1900, 14–17; 1900–01, 13–17 (BHMC); *Seventy-Five Year History*, 93.

⁷ Burns, *Saving Lives,* 30–31.

⁸ J. Gordon Bryson, *One Hundred Dollars and a Horse: The Reminiscences of a Country Doctor* (New York: Morrow, 1965), 49–50.

⁹ "Howdy Freshmen!" *University Medical* 32 (September 1927): 10.

¹⁰ "From the Medical Department Editor," *Alcalde* 3 (November 1914): 85–87.

¹¹ David G. McComb, *Galveston: A History* (Austin: University of Texas Press, 1986), 192.

¹² Burns, "Origins and Beginnings," 1401; Seaholm, "Student Life at the University of Texas Medical Department, 1901–1941," 1, 17–18.

¹³ "Medicine, 98," *Cactus* 4 (1897), 67.

¹⁴ "Escharotics," *Cactus* 12 (1905), 404.

¹⁵ "Local Notes," *University Medical* 1 (March 1896): 259.

¹⁶ Howard R. Dudgeon, "My Recollections of the Medical Department of the University of Texas at Galveston," (transcript), 30, CHP, Series 13, Box 39, File: Student Reminiscences (BHMC); Minutes of the Medical Department Faculty Meeting, Apr. 27, 1895, cited in *Seventy-Five Year History*, 54.

¹⁷ Howard R. Dudgeon Sr., "Random Undergraduate Recollections," *Alcalde* 3 (July 1915): 856.

¹⁸ James E. Thompson, "Opening Address," *University Medical* 8 (October 1903): 4.

¹⁹ Allen J. Smith, "Some Memories of the Medical Department in the Beginning," *Alcalde* 3 (July 1915): 749.

²⁰ Catalogues of the Department of Medicine of the University of Texas, 1901–1927; William S. Keiller to R. E. Vinson, Dean's Annual Report, April 1923, CHP, Series 13, Box 39, File: "Dean's Office Records," (BHMC).

²¹ W. S. Carter to S. E. Mezes, Annual Report of the University of Texas Medical Branch, May 2, 1910; W. S. Carter to S. E. Mezes, Annual Report of the University of Texas Medical Branch, May 3, 1912, CHP, Series 7, Box 27, File: Records of the President-UT Austin (BHMC).

²² Armond Samuel Goldman to Megan Seaholm, Sept. 1, 1986 (interview transcript), 2, CHP. Series 13, Box 39, File: Faculty Memories (BHMC).

²³ Edith M. Bonnet, Diary, Nov. 7, 1922 (first quotation), Nov. 22, 1922 (second quotation), Edith Marguerite Bonnet Papers, MS 16 (BHMC).

²⁴ "Personal Hygiene as the Medical Student Lives It," *University Medical* 37 (November 1932): 10–12.

²⁵ Benjy F. Brooks to Larry J. Wygant (interview transcript), 1979, 10–11 (BHMC).

²⁶ Bob Nesbitt, "Dr. Seth Morris, Sole Member of Original Medical Faculty Here Still on Staff of Institution," *Galveston Daily News*, Dec. 6, 1940.

[27] "Junior Notes," *University Medical* 27 (May 1923): 11–13.

[28] "Learning to Deal with Life and Death: The Story of Becoming a Doctor in Texas," *Texas Medicine* 76 (May 1980): 66.

[29] *Seventy-Five Year History*, 55.

[30] Minutes of the University of Texas Board of Regents, University of Texas, May 15, 1897, 123–125, CHP, Series 7, Box 27, File: Minutes, Regents: 1881–1955 (BHMC).

[31] Cunningham later proclaimed her experiences with inequity in pay as a pharmacist in Huntsville "made a suffragette out of me." In 1915, she became President of the Texas Woman Suffrage Association (subsequently the Texas Equal Suffrage Association). At the end of her life, Cunningham is said to have chosen her own epitaph: "Born a woman, died a person." Bartee Haile, "Minnie Fish: Leader of the Suffragist Cause," *In Between* (May 1987): 7; Patricia Ellen Cunningham, "Cunningham, Minnie Fisher," *Handbook of Texas Online*, http://www.tshaonline.org/handbook/online/articles/fcu24 [Accessed Aug. 18, 2011]; Silverthorne and Fulgham, *Women Pioneers*, 66–69.

[32] Silverthorne and Fulgham, *Women Pioneers*, 129.

[33] Bonnet, "Interview," 2.

[34] Bonnet, Diary, Feb., 25, 1925.

[35] Sarah R. Jourdin to Larry J. Wygant (interview transcript), 1978, 7–8 (BHMC).

[36] Margaret M. Schroch to Larry J. Wygant (interview transcript), 1978, 6 (BHMC).

[37] Edith M. Bonnet to Larry J. Wygant (interview transcript), 1978, 6 (BHMC); Silverthorne and Fulgham, *Women Pioneers*, 110.

[38] Megan Seaholm, "Student Life at the University of Texas Medical Branch, 1942–1966," 18, CHP, Series 13, Box 39, File: Student Life, 1942–1966 (BHMC); Burns, *Saving Lives*, 289.

[39] Bonnet, Diary, May 31, 1926; "Hospital Board Accepts Women Interns Subject to Certain Restrictions," *Galveston Tribune*, Jan. 26, 1926.

[40] Mary Ellen Haggard to Megan Seaholm, Sept. 7, 1988 (interview transcript), 1, CHP, Series 13, Box 39, File: Student Life Interviews (BHMC).

[41] Seaholm, "Student Life at the University of Texas Medical Branch, 1901–1941," 100.

[42] William B. Sharp, "Microbiology at the Medical College," cited in *Seventy-Five Year History*, 87; George Plunkett (Mrs. S. C.) Red, *The Medicine Man in Texas* (Houston: Standard Printing, 1930), 108; Silverthorne and Fulgham, *Women Pioneers*, 147; *Seventy-Five Year History*, 150.

[43] Nina Faye Waldrop Calhoun to Larry J. Wygant (interview transcript), 1978, 6; Sister Lucia Hartgraves to Larry J. Wygant (interview transcript), 1979, 6 (BHMC).

[44] Silverthorne and Fulgham, *Women Pioneers*, 148–149.

[45] Zidella Seibel Brener to Larry J. Wygant (interview transcript), 1978, 6 (BHMC).

[46] *Seventy-Five Year History*, 297.

[47] Seaholm, "Student Life at the University of Texas Medical Department, 1901–1941," 12–13.

[48] Quotations: Silverthorne and Fulgham, *Women Pioneers*, 36; Campbell, "A Note on the First Nursing School in Texas," 50–51.

[49] Burns, *Saving Lives*, 206–211.

[50] Howard O. Smith, "The Years 1918 to 1922," 2–3, Seventy-Five Year History Research Files (cited hereafter as 75-Year), MS 15, Box 1, File: Alumni Reminiscences (BHMC).

[51] Howard R. Dudgeon Sr., "My Recollections of the Medical Department of the University of Texas at Galveston," 12, 75-Year, MS 15, Box 1, File: Alumni Reminiscences (BHMC).

[52] *Seventy-Five Year History*, 152.

[53] Goldman to Seaholm, 2.

[54] Smith, "The Years 1918 to 1922," 287.

[55] Walter B. King, Jr., "James E. Thompson: Texas' First Professor of Surgery," *Texas Medi-*

cine 64 (February 1968): 87; Burns, *Saving Lives*, 305; McComb, *Galveston: A History*, 142, 192; *Seventy-Five Year History*, 41–42.

[56] Burns, *Saving Lives*, 109, 186; *Seventy-Five Year History*, 286. Goldman quotation from "Old Red Exhibit, 2011," by the staff of the Truman G. Blocker History of Medicine Collections, Moody Medical Library, University of Texas Medical Branch, Galveston, Texas.

[57] Burns, "Origins and Beginnings," 1402; "Sophomore Notes," *University Medical* 20 (January 1916): 25; "Sophomore Notes" *University Medical* 20 (April 1916): 18–19; "Junior Pharmacy," *University Medical* 20 (May 1916): 29; "Sophomore Notes," *University Medical* 24 (May 1920): 14; "Juniorettes," *University Medical* 28 (April 1924): 3–5; *Seventy-Five Year History*, 287.

[58] "Local and Personal," *University Medical* 7 (December 1902): 85.

[59] *Cactus* 8 (1901), 82.

[60] *Cactus* 16 (1905), 404.

[61] Sophomore Notes," *University Medical* 10 (October 1905): 27.

[62] "Freshman Class," *University Medical* 8 (November 1903): 52.

[63] Seaholm, "Student Life at the University of Texas Medical Department, 1901–1941," 25–26; "Freshmen," *University Medical* 16, (January 1912): 22–23 (quotation).

[64] "Local and Personal," *University Medical* 2 (February 1897): 196.

[65] The pharmacy fraternity, Phi Delta Chi, moved with the school to Austin in 1927. Burns, *Saving Lives*, 289–299; Burns, "Origins and Beginnings," 1402.

[66] Megan Seaholm (comp.), "Fraternities: Percent of Student Population," CHP, Series 13, Box 39, File: Fraternities (BHMC); Burns, *Saving Lives*, 290–291.

[67] Burns, *Saving Lives*, 298.

[68] Mavis P. Kelsey, *Twentieth Century Doctor: House Calls to Space Medicine* (Texas A&M University Press, 1999), 71–73.

[69] "Junior Pharmacy Notes," *University Medical* 28 (April 1924): 15.

[70] "Freshman Pharmacy Notes," *University Medical* 31 (March 1927): 31.

[71] *Seventy-Five Year History*, 288.

[72] Seaholm, "Student Life at the University of Texas Medical Department, 1942–1966," 24.

[73] C. M. Phillips, "Reminiscences of Dr. C. M. Phillips, Class of 1931," 4, 75-Year, MS 15, Box 1, Folder: Alumni Reminiscences (BHMC).

[74] Jay Collie Fish to Megan Seaholm, Sept. 7, 1988 (interview transcript), 2, CHP, Series 13, Box 39, File: Faculty Memories (BHMC).

[75] Professor Hermann's long-standing feud with the fraternity over noise, liquor, and ungentlemanly conduct eventually softened to the point that in 1965, the AKKs made him their honored guest and speaker for the groundbreaking ceremonies at their new chapter house on campus. *Seventy-Five Year History*, 288.

[76] Howard O. Smith, "The Years 1918–1922," 6.

[77] Phillips, "Reminiscences," 4.

[78] "Phillips, "Reminiscences," 5; *Seventy-Five Year History*, 280.

[79] Kelsey, *Twentieth Century Doctor*, 72–73.

[80] Denton A. Cooley to William H. Kellar, Dec. 14, 2004 (interview transcript in possession of W. H. Kellar). See also James Oates, "A History of Alpha Theta Chapter," *The Centaur* 56, No. 3 (1951), 229. Brief information concerning UTMB fraternity chapter houses can be found in "Medical Fraternity History Questionnaires," 75-Year, MS 15, Box 1, File: Fraternities-Medical (BHMC).

[81] Burns, *Saving Lives*, 299.

[82] Haggard to Seaholm, 1–2; Seaholm, "Student Life at the University of Texas Medical Department, 1901–1941," 80.

[83] Burns, *Saving Lives*, 206–208.

[84] Seaholm, "Student Life at the University of Texas Medical Department, 1942–1966," 22–23, 67–68.

[85] Seaholm, "Student Life at the University of Texas Medical Department, 1901–1941," 79, 87–88; Seaholm, "Student Life at the University of Texas Medical Department, 1942–1966," 70.

[86] Seaholm, "Student Life at the University of Texas Medical Department, 1901–1941," 89–91.

[87] Seaholm, "Student Life at the University of Texas Medical Branch, 1942–1966," 13–14.

[88] Fish to Seaholm; Dan C. Allensworth to Meagan Seaholm, Sept. 27, 1988 (interview transcript), 1, CHP, Series 13, Box 39, File: Faculty Memories (BHMC); Burns, *Saving Lives*, 299–300.

[89] *Seventy-five Year History*, 329.

[90] Minutes, UT Board of Regents, Sept. 10, 1949; Sept. 3, 1950; and Sept. 29, 1950.

[91] Goldman, Interview, 5.

[92] Burns, *Saving Lives*, 290–291.

[93] Cindy George, "UTMB Carries on Heritage to Produce More Minority Doctors," *Houston Chronicle*, Mar. 6, 2010; Burns, *Saving Lives,* 290–291; *Seventy-Five Year History*, 329.

Chapter 5

[1] Chester R. Burns, "Medical Research," *Handbook of Texas Online*, http://www.tshaonline.org/handbook/online/articles/smmrj [Accessed April 14, 2012].

[2] Chester R. Burns, "University of Texas Medical Branch at Galveston," *Handbook of Texas Online*, http://www.tshaonline.org/handbook/online/articles/kcu29 [Accessed April 14, 2012].

[3] Fish to Seaholm, Sept. 7, 1988.

[4] John A. Rhebergen, "Rehabilitation of the Ashbel Smith Building, University of Texas Medical Branch, Galveston, Texas," CHP, Series 9, Box 31, File: Old Red (BHMC); Speck, *Landmarks of Texas Architecture*, 40.

[5] Helen Smith, "Old Red: A Landmark in Texas History," *In-Between* 131 (July 1982): 21–22.

[6] "The Medical Center and Carla—A Report," CHP, Series 4, Box 13, File: Community: Hurricanes and Their impact, (BHMC); "John Sealy was Well Organized," *Galveston Daily News*, Sept. 14, 1961, 10; Stan Blazyk, "Lessons Learned and Not Learned from Carla," *Galveston Daily News*, Sept. 7, 2011.

[7] Quotation: Lillian E. Herz, "Talk of End for Old Red Brick Building Sad News," *Galveston Daily News*, Feb. 11, 1962; Smith, "Old Red: A Landmark In Texas History, 21–22.

[8] McComb, *Galveston: History*, 197.

[9] McComb, "Galveston as Tourist City," 356–357.

[10] Peter Brink to Mary Margaret Love, Sept. 12, 1980 (interview transcript), 7–8 (GTHC).

[11] McComb, *Galveston: A History*, 199.

[12] The other two buildings that once housed an entire medical school at their respective campuses are the Old Medical College Building (1835) constructed in Augusta, Georgia, and the original medical school building for the University of Louisville School of Medicine (1893), in Louisville, Kentucky. Chester R. Burns, "The Historical Significance ad Future Value of the Ashbel Smith Building—'Old Red'," *Bookman* 6 (March 1979): 1–2.

[13] Two other Galveston structures, Ashton Villa and Open Gates also received National Register honors that year. Helen Smith, "Marker Dedication of 'Old Red' Tuesday," *Galveston Daily News*, Nov. 16, 1969; McComb, *Galveston: A History*, 198. Chester R. Burns, "The Historical Significance and Future Value of the Ashbel Smith Building—'Old Red.'"

[14] Townsend quotation from "Old Red Exhibit, 2011" at BHMC.

[15] "'Save Old Red' Campaign May Determine Outcome," *Galveston Daily News*, Nov. 16, 1971; Kathleen M. Stephens, "Old Red: A Legacy Lives On," *Texas Medicine* 82 (April 1986): 51 (quotation).

[16] Wyatt C. Hedrick Architects and Engineers, Inc., "University of Texas Medical School Building, The Ashbel Smith Building, 914–916 Strand, Galveston, Galveston County, Texas," CHP, Series 9, Box 31, File: "Old Red" Building Survey (BHMC); "Old Red: A Heritage Preserved," *Horizons* 13 (Fall 1981): 26.

[17] Quotation: E. Burke Evans, "Preserving the Past," *University Medical* 4 (September 1972): 15; "Rehabilitation of the Ashbel Smith Building," 5.

[18] Chauncey D. Leake, "Preservation: A Must," *University Medical* 4 (September 1972): 17.

[19] "Old Red Receives Preservation Boosts," *The Saccarappa* 12 (December 1978): 1–2; Burns, *Saving Lives*, 123–125.

[20] Burns, "The Historical Significance and Future Value of the Ashbel Smith Building—'Old Red'," 2–3.

[21] Jan Hardin, "Money Troubles: Ashbel Smith Building or where is Old Red headed?" *Galveston Daily News*, July 4, 1976.

[22] "Old Red: A Heritage Preserved," 27; University of Texas Medical Branch, "Old Red, Old Red" (campaign brochure), 4–5, CHP, Box 31, File: Old Red (BHMC).

[23] "Old Red Receives Preservation Boosts," 1–2; "UT Regents Approve 'Old Red' Restoration," *Galveston Daily News*, June 24, 1982; Burns, *Saving Lives*, 124; Stephens, "Old Red: A Legacy Lives On," 52.

[24] Burns, *Saving Lives*, 124 (quotation). "Restoration and Dedication of a Landmark," *Galveston Daily News*, April 10, 1986; Stephens, "Old Red: A Legacy Lives On," 52–53.

[25] Masters quotation from "Old Red Exhibit, 2011" at BHMC.

INDEX